GOOD NIGHT'S SLEEP

"Straightforward, concise, and readable...will help sufferers identify and deal with sleep problems."
—*Library Journal*

"Informative...a solid, discriminating overview of the current state of knowledge on sleep...thorough, comprehensible."
—*Kirkus Reviews*

"Makes use of recent breakthroughs in sleep research to help the reader identify the troublesome sleep difficulty and select a specific program for self-treatment. Unlike other 'self-help' books for insomniacs, it takes the reader through a self-diagnostic process and then suggests remedies geared to their *specific* sleep problem."
—*Psychiatric Institute Newsletter*

"Helpful exercises and proven methods of overcoming wakeful nights."
—*Houston Chronicle*

About the Author

Jerrold S. Maxmen, M.D., is a psychiatrist in private practice in New York City, and associate professor of clinical psychiatry at the College of Physicians & Surgeons of Columbia University. He graduated from Detroit's Wayne State University School of Medicine, interned at San Francisco's Mount Zion Hospital, and took his psychiatric residency at Yale University. He taught at Dartmouth College and the Albert Einstein College of Medicine before becoming Columbia University's Director of Psychiatric Training. The author of two previous books, *Rational Hospital Psychiatry* and *The Post-Physician Era*, he was awarded a National Fund for Medical Education Fellowship and has been the Distinguished Psychiatric Lecturer of the American Psychiatric Association.

A GOOD NIGHT'S SLEEP

JERROLD S. MAXMEN, M.D.
College of Physicians & Surgeons of Columbia University

A Step-by-Step Program for Overcoming Insomnia and Other Sleep Problems

WARNER BOOKS

A Warner Communications Company

WARNER BOOKS EDITION

This Warner Books Edition is published by arrangement with
W. W. Norton & Company, Inc., 500 Fifth Avenue, New York,
N.Y. 10110

Cover design by Don Puckey

Warner Books, Inc.
666 Fifth Avenue
New York, N.Y. 10103

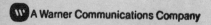 A Warner Communications Company

Printed in the United States of America

First Warner Books Printing: September, 1986

10 9 8 7 6 5 4 3 2 1

To my parents, Harold and Ethel

To my parents, Harold and Ethel

Contents

Acknowledgments

Dr. Peter Hauri has a special gift for making the unknown worth knowing, and it was his enthusiasm about sleep that first got me interested in the subject. Along the way Dr. Edward Sachar's support was instrumental in my being able to complete this project. Though I take full responsibility for any errors or omissions, Drs. Neil Kavey and Boris Rubinstein's thoughtful comments on portions of this manuscript proved invaluable.

I would like to thank my editors, Mr. Starling Lawrence and Ms. Mary Cunnane, for their patience, encouragement, and professionalism. I extend my genuine appreciation to Ms. Angela Stio for her secretarial contributions and to the staff of the New York State Psychiatric Institute's sleep laboratory, especially to Mr. Ray Goetz, Ms. Ginger Krawiec, Ms. Judy Bianca, and Dr. Joaquim Puig-Antich. Finally, there are my patients. They have taught me a great deal about sleep. But more important, by sharing those special intimacies of their lives, they have afforded me a special privilege. More than anybody else, they stimulated me to write this book. Credit is certainly due to my best and most honest critic, my wife, Mimi.

Author's Update

Since the original publication of *A Good Night's Sleep*, two widely prescribed sleeping pills have appeared: Restoril (temazepam) and Halcion (triazolam). Since they belong to the same chemical class (benzodiazepines) as Dalmane (flurazepam), they exhibit most of Dalmane's effects described in Chapter 9. Yet given that Dalmane, Restoril, and Halcion have become the three most commonly used hypnotics, respectively, the few major differences between them deserve mention.

Before doing so, four caveats: First, hypnotics are no answer to insomnia; at best, they're *temporary aids*, which should not be taken longer than three consecutive weeks. Second, no single hypnotic suits everyone; the type and dose must be *individualized*. Third, the following recommendations compare *equivalent* therapeutic doses (viz., 15 to 30 mg. for Dalmane and Restoril; 0.25 to 0.5 mg. for Halcion); higher doses for any one of these medications will change its effects relative to the others. Fourth, these are generalizations, and no one should take a hypnotic without their physician's approval.

If you want a hypnotic for one or two *nights* to *fall asleep*, Halcion is probably your best bet: It's quickly absorbed from the GI tract, reaches peak blood concentrations in one to two hours, effectively induces sleep, leaves your system quicker than the other hypnotics, and is the least sedating the next day. Dalmane is my second choice; although it's the most rapidly absorbed of all these hypnotics, it lingers longest in the body and causes the most drowsiness the following day. Restoril is the slowest to be absorbed, and more importantly, is relatively ineffective in helping people drop off.

If you want a sleeping pill for one or two *nights* to *maintain sleep*—that is, to prevent nocturnal and early-morning awakenings—then try Halcion. It effectively maintains sleep for at least a week. It also causes less hangover than Restoril or Dalmane, which are the second and third choices, respectively.

If a hypnotic is desired almost every night for two to three *weeks* to *induce sleep*, then Dalmane seems best. For up to three months, Dalmane hastens sleep and prevents nocturnal awakenings. After a week of continual use, Dalmane causes the same negligible daytime sedation as the other two hypnotics. Yet compared to Restoril or Halcion, Dalmane produces less (if any) rebound insomnia—the sleeplessness which arises five to eight days after a hypnotic is abruptly stopped. Since Restoril is poor at inducing sleep, Halcion would be my second choice.

If taken for two to three *weeks* to *maintain sleep*, Dalmane is preferred. So rapidly is Halcion eliminated from the body, that it may not be present long enough to avert early-morning awakening. Although Restoril and Dalmane equally maintain sleep and produce roughly equivalent side effects, the relative absence of rebound insomnia leaves Restoril in second position.

Which, if any, of these hypnotics is best for you depends on your idiosyncratic response and tolerance to each of them. A history of medical illness may also influence your choice: For instance, Restoril is safer for patients with *liver disease*, since unlike the other two, it is not metabolized in the liver.

A final note: Since the book's original publication, it's become abundantly clear that depression is a major cause of insomnia in children and adolescents. Depression in youth displays most of the same symptoms and therapeutic responses as major depression in adulthood (Chapter 10). Because insomnia is often the first manifestation of depression in kids, and because suicide is often becoming the last manifestation of depression in kids, recognizing these depressions is of utmost importance.

—Jerrold S. Maxmen, M.D.

CHAPTER ONE

Making a Commitment

This book has one purpose—to help you sleep. When you complete this program, you will be able to get a good night's sleep.

If you're skeptical, I can't blame you. Everywhere you go, the media, well-intentioned friends, and self-help books offer a myriad of instant cures for sleeplessness:

• For only $89.95 you can own this scientifically designed instrument which emits soothing sounds of sea waves lulling you to sleep.
• Eat asparagus tips; you will sleep like a log.
• Just list twenty-seven famous people whose last name begins with *A*, and you will promptly drift off to sleep.
• While languishing in bed, name forty instant cures for insomnia and bore yourself to sleep.

These instant cures do help some people. But the chances are that you have already gone through a litany of these quick solutions and magic gimmicks. If they had worked by now, you would not be turning to this book.

Mind you, I have nothing against instant cures. If a problem can be remedied simply, why complicate matters?

That is why some of those techniques with proven effectiveness are presented in Chapter 4. Moreover, in case you are unfamiliar with those instant cures, it would be useful for you to try them. They have worked for others; they may work for you.

This book, however, has been written specifically for people whose sleep problems have *not* been solved by instant cures. Overcoming insomnia, especially if it has been persistent, cannot be done overnight. It is discouraging enough to be plagued by insomnia. It is doubly discouraging to try remedies that repeatedly fail. When that happens, it just reinforces the notion that your problem is hopeless.

I want you to succeed. But if you don't follow this program as outlined, the chances of this happening will be substantially diminished. If you're going to skip around this book haphazardly, I'd really prefer that you not even begin. The last thing you need is another disappointment; the last thing I need is for someone to go around saying this program is a flop.

The program works, but only if you make a *firm commitment* of *time, effort,* and *patience.* Whether you choose to make this commitment is up to you. Certain things in life are within your power; others are not. Fortunately, committing yourself to this program *is* within your power. But doing so necessitates that you make a conscious and deliberate choice.

If you are inclined to make this commitment—and I hope that you are—*don't*—at least not yet. So far all I have told you in very general terms is that a firm commitment of time, effort, and patience is required. Beyond that you really don't know what the commitment specifically entails. To insure that you will not make a premature commitment, this chapter delineates the principles on which this program is based and what will be expected of you in order to complete it. Once you have this information, you will be able to make an informed commitment.

Principles and Commitments

It is 2:00 A.M. I've been awake for three interminable hours. For months I have dreaded the thought of going to bed and lying there obsessed with the idea of falling asleep. I've tried lying on my back, my stomach, my right side and then my left. I've tried lying straight as a board or curled up like a snail. I've used one pillow or several, stuffed with foam or with feathers, supporting my head or snuggled under my arm—nothing helped. I even tried counting sheep; but by the time I reached eighty-two, I was more awake than before. The whole thing is ludicrous and, yes, even embarrassing. How could I ever have become so preoccupied with getting a simple snooze?

Every time I'm just about to drop off, it seems that a honking car disrupts my tranquility, and I have to start all over again. Although every little sound disturbs me, silence is even more unbearable. I feel so alone.

I tried all the gimmicks friends suggested: concentrated on the blackness behind my eyeballs, named everyone in my high school class, imagined floating on a soft, fleecy cloud. Nothing worked.

Two months ago my doctor gave me a sedative. Initially it helped. But after several weeks, two and then three pills were necessary. Now my insomnia is as bad as ever. Should I add a fourth pill?

Maybe I should get a new mattress. Maybe it's something I ate. Maybe I'm feeling guilty about something. Maybe I really don't want to sleep. Maybe I'm neurotic.

Maybe I'm taking this all too seriously. But then, how will I ever get through tomorrow? I glance at the clock; it's 2:05 A.M. Four hours till sunrise. If only I could get even a little rest. There must, just must be a way.

Well, there is a way. There is also a catch; namely, that you have to live with and resolve this problem *by yourself*. Practically, you and you alone will have to implement this book's instructions. Emotionally, you will have only yourself to commiserate with. Do not expect sympathy or pity from others; regardless how well intentioned, neither spouses, friends, nor physicians will show much concern. Although during a long sleepless night you may wish to awaken and be consoled by your bedmate, there are limits to how much of a pest you should make of yourself. If you wear a patch over your eye, a brace around your neck, or a cast on your foot, you immediately elicit condolences. Without saying a word, people acknowledge your discomfort. On the other hand, the insomniac agonizes in private. The first time he tells friends about his sleeplessness, he gets a few suggestions along with the usual obligatory commiserations. The second time he tells them, they yawn, change the subject, walk away, or tell him to see a doctor. When he sees the doctor, the physician usually scribbles a prescription and whisks him out the door. Even the most loving spouse and devoted friends can profess concern for only so long. Wishing—nay expecting—others to be more sympathetic will not help *you* sleep any better. Focusing all your energies on what others could or should do only detracts from seeing what you can do. Ultimately, you have no choice but to "go it alone." Only you experience the sleeplessness; only you can provide the necessary emotional support; only you can rectify the problem.

Once you are prepared to "go it alone," you have made the *first major commitment*. When you assume responsibility for your own care, you also acquire a new freedom. Because you can overcome insomnia by yourself, you are no longer dependent on others for a solution. That does not mean that you should shun all available support and assistance—the more the better. But look on that additional help as a bonus, not as a necessity. By conquering insomnia on your own you become its master and not its victim—and that is freedom.

Although you will have to "go it alone," in another

respect you are hardly alone. Over half the adult population experiences a significant sleep problem at some time during their lives. Tonight, while you are desperately attempting to sleep, more than one out of every three people will be sharing your frustrations. Though feeling a kinship with 64 million suffering American adults may not be much of a consolation, at least you should know that sleeplessness is part of the human condition. It is just because it has always been part of the human condition that insomnia has largely been ignored and not taken seriously by doctors and scientists— at least not until recently.

Modern breakthroughs by sleep researchers, combined with current advances in medicine and psychology, afford today's insomniac benefits that did not exist as recently as a decade ago. Old wives' tales are charming, and fads are amusing; but they don't work. You need something that does work. For that reason this book presents only techniques that have been scientifically proven to be effective. You deserve nothing less.

You also deserve to have a basic scientific understanding of sleep problems and their cures. You should know what you are doing and why you are doing it. Although this book avoids the use of jargon, when it is occasionally necessary to employ technical terms, I have (I trust) explained them clearly. I have also refrained from using popular euphemisms. To make self-help books more palatable, many authors resort to phrases like "problems in living" when they actually mean "mental illness." Though only a few cases of insomnia are due to mental illness, at times psychiatric disorders are responsible. In the unlikely circumstance that your sleeplessness is caused by a mental illness, then you need to know that, in order to obtain proper therapy. Employing euphemisms or ignoring sensitive topics will not help your insomnia, nor will it enhance your understanding of it. Therefore, the *second major commitment* requested of you is to become *knowledgeable* about the reasons and remedies for sleeplessness.

Note that I said the "reasons and remedies" and not the "reason and remedy" for sleeplessness. Writers as well as scientists have long recognized that there are many forms of insomnia. F. Scott Fitzgerald observed, "It appears that every man's insomnia is as different from his neighbor's as are their daytime hopes and aspirations." Because there are *many causes* and *types* of insomnia, you must know what is responsible for your particular kind of insomnia, even if it's only to know that you suffer from the nonspecific type, meaning there *is* no known cause. To do so requires a *third major commitment* on your part—namely, performing the *self-assessment* in Chapter 3. By doing so you will be able to determine the exact type of sleep problem you have.

Discovering what causes your insomnia is one thing; doing something about it is quite another. We all become accustomed to behaving in certain ways and are reluctant to change. I once requested a patient of mine who was complaining bitterly of insomnia to refrain from drinking coffee after 6 P.M. "I can't do that," she exclaimed. "Take away anything—my arms, my legs—but not my coffee." In having to choose between coffee and sleep, she had to decide if change was more disturbing than insomnia. Sometimes the change is not even distressing, but "simply" requires adopting and sticking to new habits. For some of you progressive relaxation exercises will be prescribed twice a day. Performing those exercises will necessitate an alteration of your daily routine. Although it constitutes only a small change, it is a change nonetheless. Change is never easy, but, then again, neither is living with insomnia. If you really wish to get a good night's sleep, then you should be *prepared to change*, thereby fulfilling the *fourth major commitment*.

The most frequent obstacle to change is probably a lack of patience and persistence. Whether it is a program to lose weight, stop smoking, become physically fit, or vanquish insomnia, people begin with hope and determination. But during the ensuing weeks or months, this initial enthusiasm and dedication start to wane, and many people give up. The failure to maintain a program—and therefore to reap the full benefits from it—occurs for three major reasons.

First, people *rationalize*. They provide themselves with a

convenient alibi to justify breaking the program. "I'm just not in the mood to exercise today." "So what if I have a pizza; one time won't matter. I'll eat less tomorrow." "I've been so good, I deserve a cigarette." To succeed in this program you must be sufficiently honest with yourself to know when you're rationalizing.

Second, people become *discouraged*. If positive results are not attained when expected, then an attitude of "what's the use?" sets in. Not everyone benefits from a program at the same pace. Some can shed ten pounds in a week; others require three months. What is important is that the pounds are lost. Giving up prematurely is understandable, but regrettable. Although there are countless remedies for insomnia, you need only one. If the first three recommendations fail, don't lose any sleep over it; try the fourth. When asked what he was going to do in a crisis, British Prime Minister Benjamin Disraeli explained, "I suppose to use our national motto, 'something will turn up.'" If you become discouraged, remember Disraeli's motto. This program *works;* be patient and stick with it.

Paradoxically, the third reason for failure is generated out of success. After one has gone to all the effort of breaking negative habits, acquiring new skills, and apparently being well on the road to solving the problem, *overconfidence* develops. "Now that my weight is under control, a little cheating won't hurt." "I haven't smoked in two months; one cigarette won't matter." "I've got this relaxation technique down pat; I don't have to keep it up—at least not every day." Compared to the previously mentioned rationalizations, excuses based on overconfidence are more insidious. Inevitably, everybody is susceptible to believing that a transitory success is an enduring accomplishment. You be confident, not overconfident. The greatest stumbling block to permanent success is not the lack of determination in starting a program, but rather the failure to follow through with it. Thus, the *fifth major commitment,* the willingness to be *patient* and *persistent,* is a vital, and perhaps the most difficult, prerequisite for overcoming insomnia.

Because there are many kinds of sleep problems, no

single treatment is suitable for everyone. If you have a fever, it may be due to any number of ailments. You would expect a doctor to prescribe medication that specifically cures your particular illness. The same principle should apply to alleviating insomnia. Consequently, whereas many books present only a single approach to overcoming insomnia, the recommendations advanced in this book have been carefully tailored to resolve your own special sleep problem. For that reason, this book is designed to be used in various ways, depending on what your particular sleep difficulties happen to be.

The advice you'll receive will be *practical*. One author on sleep advocates that the insomniac's bedroom, including his window shades, be green, because green is relaxing and comforting to the eyes. How you can see a soothing green decor with your eyes closed escapes me, and I think it would be ludicrous to repaint your entire bedroom. The solutions set forth in this book can be readily implemented and are eminently practical.

Any method that is safe and helps you sleep is fine with me. Except for the principles outlined here, I have no axes to grind. For example, my preference is that you sleep without medication. Later you will see how sleeping pills more often aggravate than alleviate insomnia. Nevertheless, if taken judiciously, sleeping pills can be helpful. Most self-help books about insomnia zealously denounce any use of medication. Consequently, they avoid offering appropriate guidelines for people who are going to use sleeping pills anyway. I have taken an alternative approach. I will present both natural and chemical sleep-inducing methods. Which method you choose will be left up to you. But in helping you make that choice, my advice will derive from scientific data rather than from other ideological considerations. I am not interested in telling anyone how to conduct his or her life. After all, it's *your* life. However, I do want you to know the consequences of what you are doing. For instance, if you are taking marijuana in order to sleep, I would like you to understand how it will influence your sleep, both positively and negatively. Avoiding the discussion of drugs—

legal or illegal—will not prevent you from using them. As St. Augustine warned, "He who conceals a useful truth is equally guilty with the propagator of an injurious false-hood." Books that exclusively advocate natural sleep tech-niques often deny their readers vital information. As a result, in order to find out how these drugs really affect your sleep, you are stuck with relying on myths and rumors. I prefer to offer you accurate information. In giving it to you, I trust you to act wisely.

In order to be effective the remedies delineated in this program should be followed *carefully* and *systematically.* Of course, you could use this book in any way that you like. But why place yourself at a disadvantage? The steps in this program have been deliberately arranged in a specific order. Breaking this sequence by jumping around the text will only be self-defeating. Another way to fail is to not carry out the instructions exactly as written. Where there is room for latitude, I will let you know. This program has been de-signed to maximize your chance for success. Don't spoil it by taking short cuts! If you are to pursue this program, the *sixth major commitment* I am asking of you is to be careful and systematic.

The *seventh major commitment* will be to *monitor your sleep* by filling out a *daily progress chart*. This log will be a brief report on your sleep and daytime fatigue. By complet-ing this diary every day, you will at a glance be able to see your improvement and to spot any problems that might crop up. As your sleep gets better, looking at this chart will become an additional source of encouragement. My mentor Dr. John Dorsey was fond of saying, "We need all the credit we can get." Forget modesty. I want you to take pride in your accomplishments. You'll deserve it.

The final and *eighth major commitment* is to be prepared to devote sufficient *time* to the program. How much time? It's hard to say; it depends on your kind of sleep problem. Nevertheless, the following guidelines might help: (a) per-forming the self-assessment will take ten minutes; (b) de-pending on what this evaluation reveals, your tailored treat-ment program will require from one to twelve weeks to complete; (c) implementing the remedies in this program takes no more than thirty minutes a day, and frequently less than that; (d) depending on your specific type of sleeplessness, you must read four to eleven chapters (including this one); (e) filling out the daily progress chart will occupy perhaps one full minute of your time.

In terms of a time commitment, that's it. Because your time is valuable, this program consumes as little of it as possible. On the other hand, *some* time is required. But since you have a choice between wasting time agonizing over insomnia or productively spending that time doing something about it, how can you *not* afford the time to devote to this program?

Because making a commitment to this program is your first big step toward overcoming insomnia, let's quickly summarize what the commitment entails. It asks you to:

• Provide, by yourself, all of the emotional support you need, as well as to assume full responsibility for carrying out this program
• Understand the scientific reasons for the causes of and remedies for sleep problems
• Perform a self-assessment
• Change those habits, attitudes, and routines that interfere with your sleep
• Be patient and persistent in implementing the program
• Pursue the program carefully and systematically
• Maintain a daily progress chart for the duration of the program
• Devote sufficient time every day in order to guarantee a successful outcome

Now you are ready to make an informed commitment. The time and effort will be well spent, but it is *your* time and *your* effort. If you are willing to say "Yes," then let me extend to you a warm welcome.

Let's start by learning about sleep.

CHAPTER TWO

Learning about Sleep

What probing deep
Has ever solved the mystery of sleep?
—Thomas Bailey Aldrich

As a nineteenth-century poet, Aldrich was perfectly justified in posing this rhetorical question. But by "probing deep," scientists have discovered more about sleep during the past thirty years than had been known since the first primate snoozed in slime. And although some of the "mystery of sleep" remains, much of it has been solved. As the beneficiary of these insights, you inherit opportunities for overcoming sleeplessness that were completely unavailable to the legions of frustrated insomniacs preceding you.

This chapter presents an overview of the major recent advances in sleep research. Because the scope and complexity of modern sleep investigations boggle the mind, this chapter will be neither comprehensive nor detailed. Instead, it will deliberately focus on information about sleep that pertains specifically to the remedies elucidated in this book. In order to save time, many rich details will not be explored. If you wish to pursue these details, consult the bibliography in Appendix C.

In the meantime, do not overlook the fact that every day new discoveries are made, recent discoveries are revised, and old discoveries are invalidated. Because modern sleep research is technically complex, highly competent investigators often reach contradictory conclusions. But this chapter will present only generally agreed upon results. These "facts," however, are inevitably tentative. Like styles in art, facts in science continually change. Like good art, good science reveals the obvious to be illusory. Like illuminating art, penetrating science makes the unknown worth knowing about. And perhaps the best place for getting to know about sleep is in the sleep laboratory. Let's go inside and take a look.

The Sleep Laboratory

The staff of a sleep laboratory studies sleep and helps insomniacs. For their investigations researchers often seek volunteers, paying them about ten dollars a night for participating. So the next time your boss says, "You think anybody is going to pay you to sleep?" you'll know otherwise. If you're interested in picking up a few extra dollars and, more important, contributing to our knowledge of sleep, which will help millions of your fellow insomniacs, contact the staff at a local university sleep lab to see if they are looking for volunteers. (Appendix A contains a list of the major clinical sleep laboratories in North America.)

In addition to their research, the personnel of most sleep laboratories provide diagnostic and treatment services. Needlessly worried that some dreadful affliction will be unearthed, insomniacs are often reluctant to obtain the thorough evaluation that can be offered only in a sleep lab. These concerns are unwarranted. Believe me, your fantasies of what could be wrong will far exceed whatever could be discovered. Repeatedly I see patients who are surprised and relieved to find out in a lab that their sleep is perfectly normal. At times, however, a specific sleep disorder (e.g., narcolepsy) is fortunately uncovered. I say "fortunately," because knowing what the exact problem is can spare you ineffective and possibly even harmful treatment provided by otherwise good physicians who lack the specialized knowledge of the sleep expert. Furthermore, a sleep disorder does not vanish because it goes undiagnosed; whether identified or not, its symptoms remain with you. If you have a sleep disorder, you might as well know it and have it rectified by topnotch professionals. Supposing, then, that you do yourself a favor and go to a sleep disorders clinic; what should you expect?

A typical sleep disorders clinic is a peculiar hybrid—half laboratory, half bedroom. The essence of the clinic is two adjacent and strikingly different rooms. The centerpiece of the control room is the *polysomnograph*, a large space-aged device that monitors, amplifies, converts, and records numerous electrical impulses from the sleeper's muscles, eyes, and brain. This polysomnograph sprouts a dozen tentaclelike ink pens that scribble on chart paper flowing continuously at the rate of twenty-four inches a minute. During a single evening a thousand feet of tracings will accumulate.

The polysomnograph produces at least three types of recordings: the *electroencephalogram* (EEG), which indicates the brain's electrical activity or "brain waves"; the *electromyogram* (EMG), which transcribes minute electrical currents emanating from muscle fibers; the *electrooculogram* (EOG), which charts eye movements. Samples of these tracings are displayed in Figure 2.1. When used in conjunction with other instruments, the polysomnograph can also, if need be, monitor the patient's heartbeat, breathing rate, body temperature, and so forth. A tape recorder, computer terminal, blood chemistry analyzer, and other technical equipment may be in the control room as well.

Amid this technological paraphernalia is a highly trained "polysomnographic specialist"—let's just call him a "technician." Having received specific instructions from the clinic's director, the technician monitors the entire evening's activities. He makes sure that you feel at home and that the

FIGURE 2.1
POLYSOMNOGRAPHIC RECORDINGS

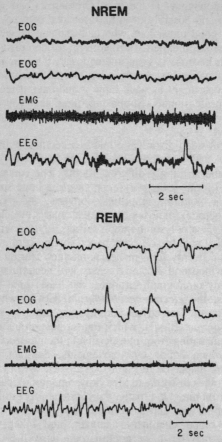

To determine the particular sleep stage, the technician notes the different characteristics produced in each of these tracings. For example, in the EMG tracing, the sharp decrease in muscle tension helps to identify REM sleep.

equipment works. In the control rooms of some sleep laboratories, he is able to see, hear, and communicate with you through a one-way mirror and a two-way intercom.

Next door to the cold, technological beehive of the control room is a warmly lit bedroom with a plush carpet, a comfortable bed, decorative furnishings, and an adjoining lavatory. The room is temperature controlled, soundproof, and pitch-dark when the lights are extinguished. The bedroom usually has all the appeal of a Howard Johnson motel suite, if that's to your taste. Certainly, every effort has been taken to make it conducive to sleep.

When you arrive at the clinic, the technician puts you at ease, shows you around, and explains what is to happen. An hour prior to bedtime he cleans with acetone or alcohol those portions of your scalp and facial skin on which the electrodes will be placed. The electrodes, which are tiny metal disks, are then applied with tape or glue to the head, chin, and next to both eyes. Those attached to the head transmit brain waves to the EEG; those attached to the chin transmit muscle tension to the EMG; those attached next to the eyes detect eye movements for the EOG. For the sake of mobility and comfort, all the wires connected to these electrodes are gathered together like a ponytail. The technician inserts these wires into a small metal box attached to the headboard of the bed. A cable travels from this box into the control room, where it is plugged into the polysomnograph. The technician double-checks the entire hookup and bids you good night. When you awake the following morning, he will be there, bleary-eyed, to greet you.

Despite all the wires, polysomnographic recordings have never harmed anyone. If a fuse goes, you won't be electrocuted. All the electrical activity goes from you to the polysomnograph, and *not* vice versa. You can easily move about, go to the bathroom, and toss and turn to your body's delight. Although mildly annoying, the electrodes will not interfere with your sleep. The technician wants you to feel comfortable not only for your sake, but also for the sake of acquiring the most accurate sleep recordings possible. There-

fore, should you suddenly feel "panicked" or "trapped,"
you may simply disconnect the wires at any time.

All the attempts to establish a homey atmosphere not
withstanding, the sleep clinic is, at least initially, a strange
environment. The tensions created by being in an unfamiliar
place can alter sleep and polysomnographic recordings of it.
The first night in the clinic is thus devoted to acclimating
you to the lab and to obtaining baseline readings. During the
second and third nights more accurate tracings are secured.
The evaluation of insomnia usually requires three evenings
in the lab; for the diagnosis of some sleep problems, however, a single night suffices.

The polysomnographic recordings are used, together with
the detailed history previously given to the clinic's sleep
expert, to analyze your difficulty. Subsequently, the clinic
staff will discuss their findings with you and suggest treatment.

By now you might be wondering what brain waves, eye
movements, and muscle tension have to do with sleep. What
can the sleep expert learn from scanning pages of scribbles?
The answer to this riddle began to unfold in 1952—the time
of *the* breakthrough.

The Breakthrough

Can you imagine anybody eager to spend hours watching
the eye movements of sleeping infants? I can't. Fortunately,
a University of Chicago graduate student felt otherwise.
Under his mentor, Dr. Nathaniel Kleitman, this graduate
student's alert observation triggered the breakthrough that
revolutionized sleep research.

As the dean of American sleep investigators, Dr. Kleitman
had searched extensively to understand sleep. In 1937 he
and Dr. B. H. Richardson spent thirty-two continuous days
sequestered in the dank recesses of Kentucky's Mammoth
Cave trying to determine if man could, in almost complete
isolation from the outside world, adjust his sleep to conform
to a twenty-eight-hour day. Out of the cave and back in the
laboratory, Dr. Kleitman pored over any clue that might

eventually pay off. Fourteen years slid by. During this time his findings were substantial, but not electrifying. Kleitman and other sleep researchers generally believed that sleep was a uniform state characterized by relative behavioral and biological inactivity. Moreover, as Kleitman himself wrote in 1939, "dreaming is present most of the time." But within a few years all of these assumptions were invalidated.

In 1952 Dr. Kleitman became intrigued by the slow, rolling eye movements that occurred when people fell asleep. Because he was interested in the more general topic of peaceful and restless sleep among infants, he wanted to know if these eye movements related to the quality or depth of sleep. There was nothing special about the experiment; it was only one among many. He thus assigned the project to one of his physiology graduate students, Eugene Aserinsky. Using an EOG, Aserinsky began the experiment.

As the night began, the sleeping child's EOG displayed what had been anticipated—slow, undulating eye movements. But shortly thereafter the pens went berserk; they moved frantically up and down the graph paper. What could be wrong? Was the child all right? Was the EOG broken? Or was it not hooked up properly? By the time he tried to unravel what had gone haywire, the pens had recovered their sanity and were once again recording those slow, pendular eye movements. As the minutes passed, Aserinsky must have wondered if he was dreaming; but if it was a dream, it was recorded on paper.

Thirty minutes of slow eye movements elapsed while Aserinsky pondered the situation. Was this merely an accident? Would it happen again? It did. Suddenly the ink pens ran amok. This was no dream; the machine was functioning properly. Staring into the child's eyes, he could see them darting back and forth beneath the closed eyelids. He could hardly believe what he was seeing. Throughout the rest of this bewildering April night, the EOG recordings alternated between relative quiescence and frenetic activity.

Any thought that this particular infant was a physiological freak vanished quickly. Everybody tested in the laboratory, adults and children alike, demonstrated this regular cyclic pattern. The frenzied oscillations soon became known as *rapid eye movements* (REMs), and the sleep accompanying them as *REM sleep*. The remaining portion of sleep, during which the eyes undulate slowly or are relatively immobile, was named *non-rapid eye movement sleep* or *NREM* (pronounced "non-REM") *sleep*.*

Aserinsky and Kleitman also noticed that body movements varied depending on whether subjects were in REM or NREM sleep. During REM sleep muscles were paralyzed, except for those involved in breathing, small facial twitches, and REMs. The person could not move even if the brain transmitted a signal to do so. On the other hand, if such a message was sent from the brain during a NREM period, the sleeper moved. Because these signals occur infrequently during NREM sleep, however, the body was usually immobile. But when the body did toss about at night, it did so in NREM and not in REM sleep. Aserinsky and Kleitman also found different breathing patterns. Whereas in REM sleep respiration was fast and irregular, in NREM sleep it was slow and regular.

Thus, sleep was *not* a uniform state. Rather, it consisted of two alternating phenomena. During NREM episodes quiescent eyes and slow, regular breathing were accompanied by infrequent bodily movements, while during REM episodes the eyes quickly glanced from side to side and breathing was fast and irregular in an otherwise paralyzed body.

For centuries prophets, poets, and scientists had tried to unlock the secret of sleep. All that time the key was, quite literally, right before their eyes. During one of your long restless nights, instead of peering enviously at your sleeping bedmate, gaze into her eyes. If you look at the right moment, you can see her eyes darting to and fro under her closed eyelids. Evolutionary data indicate that REM sleep has been present in mammals for at least 150 million years. Although these eccentric eye movements had always been

---

*Synonyms for REM sleep are paradoxical, desynchronized, or D sleep. Synonyms for NREM sleep are orthodox, synchronized, or S sleep.

there for everyone to see, it took an observant graduate student and his imaginative professor to recognize the potential importance of this bizarre activity. The breakthrough, however, had just begun.

At this juncture an energetic sophomore medical student, William Dement, joined Dr. Kleitman's team. Noting that during REM sleep the eyes darted in unison, as if the subject were awake, they speculated that the eyes might be "looking" at something—most likely a dream. Sure enough, 80 percent of the people awakened during REM periods reported dreams, whereas only 7 percent of those roused during NREM periods did so. Even subjects who emphatically denied ever having dreams, described them when awakened from REM.

Those blind since birth also dream during REM; their dreams, however, consist of sounds, not images. This observation was first made with George Shearing, the famous blind pianist, who was studied in the sleep laboratory where Aserinsky made his original discovery. Though Shearing lacked the frenzied eye movements, he did display the EEG pattern and the muscular inhibition associated with REM sleep. Those who became blind *later* in life do have visual dreams, but without rapid eye movements. In short, everybody has dreams, and they occur chiefly during the four to five REM periods of a typical night.

No longer was it tenable to view sleep as a homogeneous quiescent state. Whereas NREM periods became known as "quiet sleep," REM periods became known as "active sleep." Scientists found the latter, but not the former, to be associated with increased metabolism, faster heartbeat and pulse, higher brain and, to a lesser extent, higher body temperature, secretions of adrenal (stress) steroids, and irregular breathing. Penile erections occur in babies, children, and adults of all ages during REM but not during NREM periods.

Given the rapid eye movements, immobility of large muscles, dreams, and accelerated physiological arousal, it is as if REM sleepers possessed active brains preoccupied with vivid hallucinations but imprisoned in paralyzed bodies. REM sleepers are indeed aroused, even though they are asleep. Having many of the characteristics of wakefulness, REM sleep presents a paradox—arousal during sleep. Some researchers have even suggested that there are three, not two, natural states of consciousness: wakefulness, NREM sleep, and REM sleep.

Sleep Stages

To investigate REM and NREM sleep, Kleitman's team turned to the polysomnograph. It enabled them to discern specific sleep stages, which turned out to follow a strikingly regular pattern (Table 2.1).

If you close your eyes in a state of relaxed wakefulness, called *stage o,* the EEG shows ten ripples (or cycles) per second (Figure 2.2). This pattern, referred to as *alpha rhythm,* occurs when the mind does not need to be active, alert, or attentive; conversely, it disappears when someone yells at you, when you try to solve a problem, when you open your eyes, or when you fall asleep.

If a lack of awareness of environmental stimuli is the *sine qua non* of sleep, then you plunge rather than drift asleep. Amazingly, subjects who were dropping off while a strobe light flashed six inches in front of their open eyes became oblivious to the light at the very instant when they fell asleep. Indeed, all five senses abruptly shut down when sleep begins. (A loud noise, of course, could awaken you.)

This relative lack of sensory awareness, however, is *not* evident from the EEG recording. On falling asleep, you first descend into NREM sleep. On the EEG, alpha rhythm is gradually replaced by irregular, small scribbles indicative of *stage 1* sleep. You are calm, your thoughts meander, your muscles relax, your eyes undulate slowly, your pulse slows down, and you experience a floating sensation. As the gateway to sleep, stage 1 is so close to consciousness that you can readily be awakened from it. Indeed, if aroused during stage 1, you might insist that you were never asleep at all.

FIGURE 2.2
SLEEP EEG RECORD

**Awake
(Stage 0)**

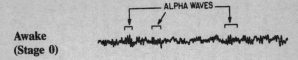

Stage 1

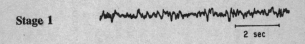

Stage 2

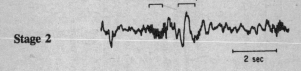

Delta Sleep

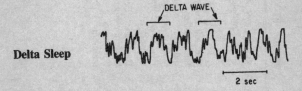

REM

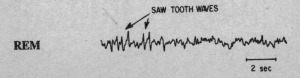

2.1 / SUMMARY OF SLEEP STAGES

SLEEP STAGE	EEG	BODILY ACTIVITY	DEPTH OF SLEEP	THOUGHT PROCESSES	MISCELLANEOUS
0 Awake	Alpha rhythm, symmetrical, 9–12 cps* waves	Slows down, decreased muscle tension	Borderline wakefulness	Relaxation, mind wanders, awareness dull	Heart and pulse rates, blood pressure, and temperature slightly diminished
1	Very small, fast, irregular, pinched waves	Eyes roll slowly on falling asleep; eyes quiescent in later stage 1 periods. Body movements slowed	Light sleep; easily awakened; might deny being asleep if awakened	Drifting thoughts and floating sensation	Temperature and heart and pulse rates decline. On occasion, may have hypnogogic hallucinations on falling asleep
2	Larger, low amplitude waves; occasional bursts of "sleep spindles" (12–14 cps waves) and "K complexes" (high amplitude waves)	Eyes quiet. Few body movements. Snoring is common	Light to moderate sleep; relatively easy to awaken with moderate intensity sounds. Eyes will not see if opened	Some thought fragments; memory processes diminished; if awakened, may describe a vague dream, but only infrequently	Decreased heart, pulse, and metabolic rates, blood pressure, and temperature; regular breathing with increased airway resistance (snoring)

3	Slow, large 1–2 cps delta waves make up 20 to 50% of EEG	Occasional movement, eyes quiescent	Deep sleep; takes louder sounds to be awakened	Rarely able to remember thoughts; a few vaguely formed dreams; possible memory consolidation	Metabolic, pulse, and heart rates, blood pressure, and temperature decrease further. Greater secretion of growth hormone
4	More than 50% delta waves	Occasional movement, eyes quiet	Deepest sleep; very difficult to awake	Virtual oblivion, very poor recall of thoughts if awoken. Possibly involved in memory consolidation	Continued decline in cardiovascular, temperature, and metabolic rates; increased secretion of growth hormone probably restores bodily tissues
REM	Irregular, small waves resembling awake EEG; bursts of "sawtooth" waves	Large muscles paralyzed; toes, fingers, and small facial muscles twitch; erections; snoring usually ceases	Variable; if sound incorporated into dream, then harder to awake	80% dreaming, good vivid dream recall, especially later in the evening. Possibly involved in unconscious conflict resolution	Heart rate 5% greater than during NREM; blood pressure and pulse, cerebral blood flow, and metabolic rates increase. Brain temperature increases. Irregular (slow and then fast) breathing; one-half extra breath a minute. Slight increase in body temperature.

*cps = cycles (waves) per second.

After several minutes in stage 1, you sink into *stage 2* NREM sleep. Spindlelike markings and *K complexes* characterize stage 2 on the EEG. (Figure 2.2) If your eyes were taped open during this stage, you would nevertheless be unable to see. Because of the diminished sense of touch, having your eyes taped open is—believe it or not—only slightly annoying. Although with somewhat more difficulty than during stage 1, you can be awakened by sounds with relative ease during stage 2. If that occurs, you may believe you were never asleep, even though you may have been dozing for ten minutes. The deeper the stage of sleep, the harder it is to be awakened. Moreover, as you descend into deeper NREM sleep, heart, pulse, and respiratory rates, temperature, and oxygen consumption decline; these changes reflect a slowing of the body's metabolism.

After twenty to forty minutes of sleep, the EEG begins to show occasional tall, slow waves each lasting a second; these so-called *delta waves* herald the onset of *stage 3*. Technically, when they occupy 20 percent of the EEG, stage 3 has officially arrived. In stage 3 you are hard to awaken, your breathing is slow and even, and your temperature, pulse, and blood pressure continue to decline.

After about ten minutes, when more than half of the EEG's tracings consist of delta waves, *stage 4* begins. Because the EEG is characterized by delta waves, stages 3 and 4 are collectively designated as *delta sleep*. While you are in stage 4, your metabolism slows and you are very difficult to awaken. Should a loud noise or an irritating alarm buzz, you will wake up, but only after a few seconds. Many children in stage 4 are virtually unarousable; even if yelled at, some children are able to wake up only after several minutes. When roused from the oblivion of stage 4, the annoyed sleeper, whether child or adult, will temporarily be confused. At this moment with the proper inclination and opportunity, you can quickly plummet back into stage 4. Although the function of delta sleep is still in doubt, it appears that these deepest of sleep stages help to restore and revitalize the body.

About forty to fifty minutes after falling asleep, you start to quickly reascend through stages 3 and 2. At this point, having concluded the evening's first NREM period (i.e., stages 1–2–3–4–3–2), you finally enter your initial REM period. While sawtooth waves appear on the EEG, vivid hallucinations appear in your mind. Unless awakened at this time, you will not remember this first dream the next morning. A kind of "coming attraction" that precedes the "feature films" to follow, this initial REM period usually lasts five to ten minutes. Approximately seventy to eighty minutes after you fell asleep, then, the first REM period ends; it marks the completion of the evening's initial NREM-REM *sleep cycle* (i.e., stages 1–2–3–4–3–2–REM).

This sleep cycle repeats itself four to five times throughout the night. Usually, the second and third cycles last 110 and 120 minutes respectively. Subsequent sleep cycles are shorter, approximately 90 minutes each. (Figure 2.3 diagrams a typical adult sequence of sleep stages throughout a night.)

FIGURE 2.3
NORMAL ADULT SLEEP STAGES

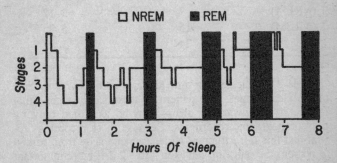

Notice on Figure 2.3 that the first half of the evening is dominated by deep, restorative delta sleep; REM episodes are few and brief. As the night proceeds, however, delta sleep is gradually replaced by lighter stage 2 sleep, while the frequency and duration of REM periods increase. The night's final REM episode typically lasts thirty to forty minutes. You may have observed this yourself; when the alarm goes off, you often awake from a dream.

In general, the typical adult spends half his night in stage 2 sleep. The other half is split about evenly between delta and REM sleep. A normal eight-hour sleeper thus dreams roughly two hours a night. Throughout that night, especially near the end of it, the sleeper may awake two to four times out of either REM or NREM stage 1 sleep. These awakenings, however, are momentary; the person immediately plunges back to sleep, without realizing he was ever awake.

2.2 / AVERAGE PERCENTAGES OF SLEEP STAGES IN ADULTS PER NIGHT

STAGE	AVERAGE	NORMAL RANGE
0 (Awake)	1	0–3
1 (NREM)	5	1–10
2 (NREM)	48	40–60
3 (NREM)	7	3–12
4 (NREM)	15	5–25
REM	24	15–35

Table 2.2 indicates the time adults usually devote to each of the sleep stages. The pattern of these sleep stages—that is, the *infrastructure* of sleep—can be identified only by polysomnographic recordings. Because these recordings reveal that this infrastructure varies tremendously from person to person, the range of values in Table 2.2 is more important than the single average figure.

Speaking of numbers, I'm about to bombard you with them. I'm sorry, but necessity calls. If you're like me, when barraged by numbers, you're tempted to flee. But because I want you to stick with and understand the following section, I've done my best to keep the numbers to a minimum.

Don't confuse averages or normality with health. The average (i.e., normal) American adult male is 5'9" tall. If someone is 6'3", his height is certainly abnormal, but he is hardly unhealthy. Health entails a sense of well-being. If the particular dimension of health is quantifiable, it usually falls within a *range of normality*. Whether you speak of height, anxiety, weight, or sleep, there is always a range of normality. It is, indeed, abnormal to be exactly normal. Therefore, in reading the following sets of figures, don't be worried if you're not precisely average. On the other hand, if your sleep falls outside the range of normality, this might be a cause for concern.

Age and Sleep

Among all the factors that naturally influence sleep, age is the most important. In reviewing the effect of age, we'll look at the infrastructure of sleep and the *total sleep time* (TST)—the number of hours you actually sleep between when you first drop off and when you finally awake in the morning. Both the infrastructure of sleep and TST vary enormously throughout the life cycle.

Newborns enter the world filled with dreams—perhaps. Premature infants, presumably those in the womb, spend up to 80 percent of their sleep in REM. Although two-thirds of newborns slumber between fourteen and eighteen hours a day, what they have to dream about for seven to nine hours each day escapes me. Of course, it is possible that a baby's REM sleep may be unaccompanied by dreams. Because the content of dreams is derived from life, what conceivable experiences do babies, especially prior to birth, have to draw upon? Therefore, whether newborns dream remains an unanswered question; they are notoriously unreliable informants.

Between the time when he swims in embryonic fluid and celebrates his six-months birthday, the infant's TST and REM sleep decline sharply. By the time the child reaches six months, he typically sleeps 13.7 hours, spending 30 percent of that time in REM.

Showing little regard for parental desires, the newborn snoozes six to eight times throughout a twenty-four-hour period. By the age of six months, the child has consolidated his sleep pattern; usually his sleep is divided between a morning and an afternoon nap, and a longer nighttime sleep. During the first six months the time the child is continuously awake expands by 40 percent (from 2.4 hours to 3.6 hours), while his longest sleep interval more than doubles (from 4.1 hours to 8.5 hours). As his pattern of sleep gradually conforms to that of his parents, the infant sleeps for increasingly longer periods at night without interruption. Whereas at two months about half of all babies awake at least once during the evening, by six months 80 percent of them sleep through the night. By this time even their parents are sleeping better.

Although REM and NREM can be differentiated clearly on the newborn's EEG, the substages of NREM sleep cannot be distinguished. By the age of two, however, NREM stages finally become organized and stabilized. From here until adolescence the sleep EEG of the child more and more resembles the adult pattern.

During the preschool years the child needs less sleep, takes fewer daytime siestas, and snoozes for longer intervals at night than previously. Among children aged two, three, four, and five, the percentage of those having a daytime nap decreases from 92, 88, 64, to 5, respectively. On the average, 20 to 25 percent of the two-year-olds, 10 percent of the three-year-olds, and 5 percent of the five-year-olds wake up at night. Thus, nighttime sleep becomes increasingly consolidated.

From the age of five until early adulthood there are very few significant changes in sleep, except for the gradual reduction in TST. By the age of twelve, the 60-minute REM-NREM cycle of childhood has been replaced by the 90 to 110-minute cycle characteristic of adulthood. Moreover, REM periods approximate the normal adult pattern of 25 percent of TST.

Childhood sleep requirements vary considerably; heaven does not ordain a fixed quantity of sleep for everyone.

Typically, German and English children sleep sixty to ninety minutes less than their American counterparts. How much a child should sleep depends on the child, and not on what is inscribed in books—including this one.

The next major sleep changes occur in the elderly. Once again, there is tremendous variability. Just as stereotypes about the aged as people are misleading, so too are stereotypes about their sleep. Typically, however, their sleep is more fragmented and variable than it was earlier in life. Table 2.3 compares the usual sleep patterns of twenty- and sixty-year-olds. Although the sleep time remains constant, the infrastructure of that sleep undergoes significant alterations. Compared to that of younger adults, the sleep of the aged is lighter and, therefore, less refreshing. The elderly show an eightfold increase in the frequency of nighttime awakenings. Nevertheless, among the aged, one out of five sleeps uninterruptedly through the evening. On the other hand, many are distressed by awakening a dozen or more times a night. Typically, the elderly have more than twice the amount of stage 1 and a third of the delta sleep of younger adults. Although the delta sleep of some of the elderly resembles that of thirty-year-olds, 25 percent of the aged have no deep sleep whatsoever. Thus, while they sleep, as long as younger adults, the elderly often believe they are sleeping less. This misperception stems from the topsy-turvy infrastructure of their sleep. Because they have

2.3 / SLEEP PROFILES OF 20- AND 60-YEAR-OLDS

	SLEEP STAGES						NUMBER OF DAYTIME NAPS	AVERAGE NIGHT SLEEP*	SLEEP TIME†	RANGE OF SLEEP TIME
AGE	0	1	2	3	4	REM				
20	1%	5%	48%	7%	15%	24%	0	7.7 hrs.	8.1 hrs.	6–9 hrs.
60	8%	12%	51%	5%	3%	21%	2/week	7.2 hrs.	8.2 hrs.	5–11 hrs.

*Nighttime sleep only.
†Total of day and nighttime sleep.

a disproportionate amount of lighter sleep, they genuinely feel that TST has diminished.

Daytime naps are common among the elderly; many seventy-year-olds snooze once or twice a day. Another striking change, especially among men, is that the *range* of their TST fluctuates more than among younger adults.

Insomnia among the elderly is pervasive. Although those under fifty complain more often about being unable to fall asleep, those over fifty are disturbed more frequently by middle-of-the-night and early-morning awakenings. Because everyone's sleep is lighter during the second half of the night, the elderly, with their propensity toward excessive stage 1 sleep, cannot possibly sleep any more lightly without waking up. Thus, they are prone to waking up early and often have difficulties relapsing into a satisfying slumber. While lying awake, they, like insomniacs of all ages, frequently work themselves into a tizzy over losing sleep. If only they would first ask themselves, "How much sleep do I *actually* need?" considerable grief might be spared.

Sleep Requirements

Social and cultural expectations have down through the centuries influenced our notions of how long we are supposed to sleep. An English proverb says, "Nature requireth five hours sleep; custom taketh seven; idleness takes nine; and wickedness eleven." Another English proverb views long-sleepers with contempt: "Six hours' sleep for a man, seven for a woman, and eight for a fool." So much for the wisdom of proverbs.

A more pervasive, but no less ludicrous, belief is that *everybody* should have eight hours of sleep. Maimonides proclaimed, "The day and night is twenty-four hours. It is sufficient for a person to sleep one third thereof, which is eight hours." Even today, children are warned that plagues and pimples will break out unless they sleep for at least eight hours. Many adults still believe that without those precious eight hours, one has a "sleep problem." Nonsense!

The idea that everyone must have the same amount of sleep—whether it's six, seven, or eight hours—is a myth. Some people function quite well with only three hours of sleep; others feel like zombies without ten hours of sleep; an Italian farmer and an Australian claim never to sleep at all.

Because sleep requirements vary, many people worry needlessly about not sleeping for eight hours. If you sleep six hours a night and are not fatigued the next day, you do *not* have a sleep problem. Instead, you are a highly efficient sleeper. Think of it this way: If you sleep six hours without being tired the following day, you have not *lost* two hours of sleep; you have *gained* two extra waking hours. From this perspective you have thirty additional days a year to pursue whatever brings you pleasure. For years a physician colleague of mine has awakened at 3 A.M. every day. Instead of fretting about insomnia, he enjoys catching up on his professional reading and writing.

The problem of all too many self-labeled "insomniacs" is not that they sleep too little, but that they worry too much. They agonize over a nonexistent sleep problem. The difficulty is in their attitude, not in their sleep. I cannot overemphasize that if you are worried about not getting sufficient sleep, even though you are not tired the next day, you have nothing to be concerned about. If you will believe me—and I hope you will—you can put your mind (and this book) to rest.

Those who require more sleep tend to be worriers; they are more likely to fret about their health and life. Short sleepers, by contrast, tend to work more efficiently and live more contentedly.

Under certain temporary circumstances sleep requirements may change. In general, the need for sleep diminishes during times of well-being, while it increases during times of disease, distress, and depression. More specifically, people sleep longer during periods of illness, weight gain, stress, unhappiness, bereavement, pregnancy, premenstruation, strenuous exercise, and unenjoyable intellectual activities. Thus sleep is frequently prolonged when you cram for an exam, lose a job, or break up an intimate relationship. On the other hand, the need for sleep declines when you lose weight or feel that "all is right with the world."

Under normal situations you only need as much sleep as is necessary to feel refreshed the following day. Typically, that calls for seven to eight hours; but *for you* it may mean four, six, eight, or ten hours. Because only you can judge if you feel rested, only you can determine your sleep requirements.

Sleep Loss

If you're fatigued as a result of insufficient sleep, what are the other effects of sleep loss? Dr. R. T. Wilkenson defined sleep loss as sleeping less than two hours on a single night or less than five hours on two consecutive nights. He showed that the performance of routine, simple, boring tasks was the first to be impaired. The disruption of more complex and less repetitive activities required greater sleep deprivation.

Obstacles to carrying out tasks, whether simple or complex, can be overcome momentarily by sufficient motivation. After a sleepless night, a tollbooth operator would have more difficulty collecting quarters than would a boxer trying to demolish his opponent. Likewise, sleep deprivation would interfere more with a student's ability to drive long distances than with his ability to take an important examination. In 1960, studies conducted in France revealed that when performing the same task, men secrete more epinephrine (adrenalin) and norepinephrine (noradrenalin) after being sleep deprived than after being well rested. Thus, quite literally, "getting the juices flowing" can compensate for impaired functioning due to sleep loss.

If substantial sleep loss continues for several days, more severe consequences may arise. In 1894, while conducting the first sleep-deprivation studies in animals, Marie de Manaceine found that puppies died when kept awake for four to six days. Humans are more resilient, but the effects of sleep loss on them can be substantial.

In 1959, as a March of Dimes fundraising stunt, thirty-two-year-old disc jockey Peter Tripp stayed awake for more than eight consecutive days. After two days of continued wakefulness, he became psychotic. He began to see an imaginary rabbit in the studio and cobwebs on his shoes. Specks on a table appeared to be bugs. By the fifth day a doctor's suit looked like a colony of furry worms. A nurse appeared to drool. Becoming increasingly paranoid, he fled from his glass-lined broadcasting booth, convinced that a (non-existent) fire had been deliberately set to test him. Day six found him unable to determine who and where he was. On the final day of this combination of experiment and fundraising, while being examined by a soberly dressed physician, Tripp felt the doctor was a funeral director who was burying him alive. Despite being plagued by conspiratorial thoughts, delusions, hallucinations, and a fading memory, he still was able, throughout the entire vigil, to broadcast his three-hour radio show so effectively that his audience was unable to detect the grotesque nightmare he was undergoing. After two hundred torturous hours, he slept. Thirteen hours later he awoke, free of all bizarre ideas and perceptions.

Compare that horror story to the tale of Randy Gardner, a sandy-haired, seventeen-year-old San Diego student who stayed awake for eleven consecutive days without experiencing any major adverse psychological effects. In 1965, as part of his high-school science-fair project, he sought to win a place in the *Guinness Book of World Records* for continuous wakefulness. Although during the day he found it relatively easy to remain awake, at night he was strongly tempted to sleep. He refused to succumb. By the fourth day, however, he had difficulty concentrating, became irritable, and briefly imagined a fog haloing the street lights. On day nine he fantasized that he was a black football hero. Occasionally his sentences became disjointed and his vision blurred. But these aberrations were few and transient. He never became psychotic, nor did he have significant problems in functioning. During the last night of his "wakeathon," he and Dr. Dement played over a hundred pinball games. Randy won every one! After 264 hours, a new Guinness world record had been set, and Randy proceeded to sleep fourteen and two-thirds hours.

Peter Tripp and Randy Gardner both stayed awake for inordinately long periods; then why did the disc jockey become floridly psychotic while the high school student did not? It may have been because Randy was younger, healthier, more physically active during his vigil, and more emotionally stable to begin with. Nobody really knows. Nevertheless, these two experiments demonstrate three important points.

First, one night of sound sleep will compensate for the most dramatic ill effects of many nights without sleep. After Peter and Randy completed their wakeathons, they slept for only about thirteen and fifteen hours respectively. Subsequently, they slept normally. They did not have to recoup hour for hour, all the sleep they had lost.

Second, after many sleepless nights it is still possible to perform tasks demanding highly developed skills. Even at the end of their vigils, Peter was effectively spinning records and Randy was victoriously shooting pinballs. Despite sleeplessness, if necessity calls, the body responds.

Third, the ability to maintain previously developed complex skills is even more remarkable given that during protracted wakefulness one simultaneously undergoes progressive psychological deterioration. Volunteers at the Walter Reed Army Institute of Research who were kept awake up to ninety-eight hours had many of Randy's and Peter's experiences. After one full day of wakefulness, the volunteers showed exhaustion, reduced powers of concentration, a proclivity for withdrawing from people, and annoying physical symptoms, such as burning or itching eyes, blurred vision, and headaches. Between thirty and sixty sleepless hours, distortions and other misperceptions of the environment occurred. The walls moved to and fro, small objects flew by out of nowhere, tables grew smaller, and a foggy halo surrounded lights. After ninety hours, vivid hallucinations and even dreams unexpectedly intruded into consciousness. Some of the volunteers suddenly laughed or grew irritable for no reason. Time expanded and contracted. Reality and fantasy became almost indistinguishable.

After twenty-four hours, the Walter Reed volunteers had lapses of attention that would under other circumstances have been attributed simply to exhaustion. Because the volunteers were being monitored, however, during these moments of inattention, their EEGs revealed that slow sleep waves were replacing normal waking EEG patterns. Although seeming to be awake, they were evidently falling asleep for two or three seconds without being aware of it. These bursts of sleep, now called *microsleeps,* probably happen more often than scientists previously recognized.

The occurrence of microsleeps might be one of the reasons that chronic insomniacs do not suffer the extreme mental deterioration displayed by the Walter Reed volunteers. Another is that, unlike the wakeathon participants, even the most severe insomniac obtains *some* sleep.

In comparison to good sleepers, poor sleepers are more apt to be anxious, depressed, worried, introverted, and hypochrondriacal. Whether these symptoms cause or result from insomnia is unknown. Anxiety leads to insomnia, and insomnia leads to anxiety. This vicious spiral escalates, producing more anxiety and more sleeplessness.

In order to interrupt this spiral, some of the remedies suggested in this book capitalize on the relationship between two concepts—*prior wakefulness* and *sleep latency.* Prior wakefulness refers to the time between the most recent awakening and falling asleep. If you arise at 8 A.M. and doze off at 11 P.M., your prior wakefulness is fifteen hours. If you followed the same schedule, but napped between 4 and 5 P.M., your prior wakefulness would be only six hours. Sleep latency is the time between going to bed and entering stage 1 sleep. When you say, "It took me forever to fall asleep," you are referring to a prolonged sleep latency.

As prior wakefulness increases, sleep latency decreases, and vice versa. If you have been awake for ten hours, it will take you, on the average, twenty-five minutes to fall asleep.

On the other hand, if you have been awake for twenty hours, it will take you about thirteen minutes to drop off.

Prior wakefulness has only a minimal effect on TST. Even though Peter and Randy were awake longer than a week, when they finally hit the sack, they slept only an additional five and seven hours respectively. Under more typical circumstances, being awake an extra five hours will lead to only an additional fifteen minutes of sleep.

Increased prior wakefulness does bring about a dramatic change, however: It leads to a higher proportion of stage 4 and fewer, if any, nighttime awakenings. Conversely, light sleep with frequent awakenings will follow a shorter period of prior wakefulness. When prior wakefulness increases, the proportion of REM diminishes slightly, probably because it has to make way for the expanded stage 4 sleep. Thus, after being awake for an extended period, the body "prefers" the deeper, more restorative stage 4 sleep over the lighter but more interesting REM sleep. It is as if the body were saying, "Invigorate first, dream later."

Dr. Wilse Webb demonstrated that if people slept two hours less for four to seven nights, they retained the same amounts of delta sleep, but lost REM sleep. When this experiment was continued for eight weeks, or when TST was reduced to four hours a night, the proportion of deep sleep increased even further. Clearly, the body is very possessive of its stage 4 sleep. This natural reluctance to relinquish delta sleep would be more understandable if *everyone* deprived of it became exhausted. But as Webb himself has cautioned, 25 to 33 percent of fifty-year-olds get along fine without any stage 4 sleep. Thus, although deep sleep serves a restorative function for many, the necessity of stage 4 is not universal.

Following protracted wakefulness the body initially recoups by grabbing stage 4 sleep, but what happens if you are deprived of stage 4? This may occur with increasing age, with the use of alcohol and some medications, as well as during medical and psychiatric illnesses. This reduction of stage 4 also can happen for no apparent reason.

Devising a method for evaluating the effect of only losing

stage 4 sleep is neither as simple nor as direct as you might imagine. In the sleep laboratory the investigator could eliminate stage 4 by arousing a subject every time he entered stage 4. If that was done, would the results only signify the loss of stage 4 or would they reflect the consequences of being awakened constantly? If the scientist used drugs that suppress stage 4, how would he know whether the findings were due solely to stage 4 deprivation or to some other effects of medication? To get around these predicaments, Drs. Robert Agnew and Wilse Webb devised a clever yet simple plan. Every time the sleeper's EEG was about to enter stage 4, a buzzer would sound. The sound was insufficient to awaken the subject, but loud enough to divert his sleep into stages 2 and 1. In this manner they could eliminate stage 4 selectively without awakening the sleeper or introducing medication.

Following a week of deprivation of stage 4, college-student subjects became mildly lethargic and depressed. At this point their sleep patterns were recorded again, but without the use of the buzzer. Not only did stage 4 return immediately, but it constituted a higher percentage of TST than before the deprivation experiment began. This phenomenon is called *stage 4 rebound;* it always occurs after stage 4 has been reduced. The greater the loss of stage 4, the greater the rebound. This rebound lasts for several days, after which the proportion of stage 4 gradually returns to normal.

Whereas losing stage 4 sleep may lead to mild depression and lethargy, being awakened every time they were about to enter REM produced in Dr. Dement's subjects anxiety, irritability, and difficulties in concentrating. Many scientists argued, however, that these symptoms arose not because REM was deprived specifically, but rather because the subjects were constantly having their sleep interrupted. To resolve this dispute, Dr. Agnew awoke one group of Florida volunteers every time they entered REM and another group every time they entered stage 4. He showed that whereas the students deprived of stage 4 became fatigued, the students deprived of REM became irritable and had more difficulties conducting social interactions. Although Agnew's investigation confirmed Dement's findings, the debate over whether REM deprivation causes psychological difficulties was anything but settled.

Dr. Gerald Vogel pointed out that patients who have taken antidepressant medication for years do not experience any adverse psychological consequences, even though these drugs virtually eliminate REM sleep. He also observed that REM deprivation without drugs actually helps some patients with severe depression. On the other hand, Dr. Ernest Hartmann, while admitting that the evidence is still inconclusive, contends that REM deprivation probably fosters anxiety and irritability, along with difficulties in concentrating and socializing. He notes that persistently removing REM by awakening subjects is nearly impossible, because after five to ten days the subjects immediately slip back into REM. By contrast, excluding REM completely for extended periods by using medications is very easy to accomplish. For these reasons he maintains that the presence of symptoms following REM deprivation may depend more on the techniques used than on the loss of REM itself. All the experts agree on one point: The once widely held belief that REM deprivation leads to madness is a myth.

Once either of the REM-depriving methods is terminated, a striking overcompensation of REM occurs. This phenomenon is known as *REM rebound*. Usually REM periods occupy 20 to 25 percent of TST. But after REM deprivation, 30 to 50 percent of TST is spent in REM. During this REM rebound, not only does the sleeper dream more frequently, but his dreams are intensely vivid, often frightening. Even without having unsettling dreams, the person is apt to awake repeatedly. Fortunately, after a week of undisturbed sleep, REM periods gradually return to normal. But if REM suppression is maintained for months, as often occurs with the use of sleeping pills, REM rebound and disturbed sleep can persist even longer.

Sleeping Pills

The quest for the ideal sleeping potion has continued for centuries. Although I would not want Iago as my pharmacist, in *Othello* he astutely observes, "Not poppy, nor mandragora,/ Nor all the drowsy syrups of the world,/ Shall ever medicine thee to that sweet sleep/ Which thou owedst yesterday."

What I find remarkable is that in our supposedly "pill-popping" society Iago's message is slowly but finally getting across. Sleep research into the effects of prescription sleeping pills—technically called *hypnotics*—has recently altered physicians' prescribing habits. Whereas from 1965 to 1969 prescriptions for hypnotics in the United States increased by 9 percent, from 1971 to 1977 they actually declined by 39 percent. In 1971 a record 41.7 million prescriptions for hypnotics were written; by 1977 this figure, despite a larger population and more aggressive marketing by pharmaceutical firms, had fallen to 25.6 million. Although this trend is encouraging, given the limited value of hypnotics, the figure of 25.6 million prescriptions remains excessive, if not frightening.

In 1980 approximately 6 percent of adults took hypnotics, and about a third of these used sleeping pills nightly. Women employed hypnotics twice as often as men did, which is roughly in line with their greater utilization of medical services. The elderly also use "sleepers" in disproportionate quantities; in 1977 those over the age of sixty consumed 39 percent of all hypnotics, even though they constituted only 15 percent of the population.

Today, Dalmane is the most widely used sleeping pill, constituting 53 percent of all prescriptions for hypnotics. Chemically, and therefore in its physiological effects, Dalmane resembles the popular tranquilizers Valium and Librium. The second most widely used hypnotics are the barbiturates, which include Seconal, Nembutal, and Tuinal. Although barbiturates presently compose 17 percent of the prescription sleeping-pill market, in 1965 they accounted for 58 percent of it. Barbiturates have been superseded by Dalmane, principally because Dalmane is less dangerous and less addictive, but also because it has a more prolonged effectiveness and causes a negligible REM rebound. Nevertheless, both Dalmane and the barbiturates create their fair share of problems.

Barbiturates, like many other hypnotics (e.g., Doriden, Quaalude, Noludar, and Placidyl), eventually disturb sleep by causing REM rebound. Although initially barbiturates effectively induce sleep, they also decrease REM. When used of the drug is stopped, REM rebound erupts with a vengeance. Frequent awakenings interrupt numerous unsettling dreams. Because delta sleep is substantially replaced by REM sleep, the evening's rest fails to refresh.

The result is that many insomniacs start taking barbiturates again. Although barbiturates temporarily bring relief by suppressing REM rebound, this comfort is short-lived. Like most hypnotics, barbiturates lose their soporific effect within two weeks of nightly use. At this point the only way to induce sleep and to control REM rebound is to increase the dose. Whereas initially a single barbiturate capsule induced sleep, in one to three months several capsules may be needed to bring it on. When the dose becomes excessive, addiction develops. If the drug is then suddenly discontinued, the patient undergoes withdrawal, which includes a massive REM rebound with disturbing dreams that intrude into consciousness.

Because the physiological effects of alcohol are akin to those of barbiturates, a similar process occurs when chronic alcohol intake is abruptly stopped or markedly diminished. The subsequent REM rebound that accompanies delirium tremens—the DTs—produces frightening dreamlike hallucinations, even while the person is awake.

Whereas barbiturates, alcohol, and most other hypnotics substantially suppress REM, Dalmane does not. If used nightly, Dalmane can induce sleep for as long as a month. For many people, however, Dalmane also produced daytime lethargy. It reduces delta sleep, and after continued use it lingers in the bloodstream for fifty to a hundred hours.

Taking Dalmane, in short, creates the very problem it seeks to avoid. Instead of being refreshed, you are apt to become fatigued by Dalmane-generated sleep. Daytime naps become irresistible. Since prior wakefulness is substantially reduced, it becomes even harder to fall asleep. Needless to say, at this point the thought of taking additional Dalmane for sleep becomes all the more tempting.

Thus, paradoxically, the *continued use of all types of sleeping pills aggravates rather than alleviates insomnia.* Hypnotics can be helpful, but only if used sparingly and episodically, not persistently.

The Sleep Environment

During World War II, while artillery fired and bombs exploded, soldiers slept in the trenches. They had every reason not to sleep, but they slept. One steamy afternoon my wife fell asleep while standing in a wretched bus rattling along a crater-infested Majorcan back road. Given that Americans spend over one billion dollars annually on mattresses, I can't help wondering how, for millennia, our ancestors slept on desert sands, in fields, and on rocks. If you're a good sleeper and tired, you can sleep anyplace, anytime. If you're a light sleeper, however, it's another matter.

The most frequent complaint about a distracting sleep environment pertains to noise. Several facts about the effects of sound on sleep are known: (a) The deeper your sleep, the louder a sound must be to awaken you. (b) The more sleep you have accumulated during the evening, the more likely you are to be awakened by a sound, even if you are in the same sleep stage. For example, you will more readily awaken from stage 2 later in the evening than you would have from stage 2 earlier on. (c) Some people are seven times more susceptible to noise-induced awakenings than others are. (d) Despite diminished hearing with age, the elderly are more prone to be awakened by sounds. (e) Women are more likely than men to have their sleep upset by noise. (f) Loud sounds are more apt to awaken you than quieter ones. (g) Softer noises having personal significance will more likely awaken you than will meaningless but louder sounds. A mother will blissfully sleep through a thunderstorm but arise instantly at the sound of her child's whimperings. (h) You are less apt to be aroused by persistent noises than by episodic changes of sound. An apocryphal story tells of a sleeping miller who, in the early 1870s, ground wheat by using a waterwheel. When the waterwheel's continuous squeaking and rumbling ceased, the silence would immediately awaken him. Not only was there a change in sound intensity, the silence also had personal significance—it meant that the waterwheel deserved attention. (i) Noise will lighten the stage of sleep. In comparison to residents of quieter neighborhoods, those living adjacent to airports show less delta and more stage 1 sleep on their EEGs; they also awaken more frequently at night.

Thus, while noise is hardly conducive to sleep, neither is silence necessary for it. Many people not only prefer to fall asleep with a radio playing; they actually claim they are unable to do so without it. Furthermore, routine noise often becomes the insomniac's scapegoat. When desperately trying to fall asleep, you may be driven up the wall by a dripping faucet. You may find, however, that after turning off the faucet, you become annoyed by honking automobiles. Once the cars go away, you may be disturbed by music from an adjacent room. Thus, in many circumstances it is not that noise of low and moderate intensity disturbs sleep, but rather that the disturbed sleeper rivets his attention on distracting noise.

Preferably, you should sleep in a room of moderate temperature—between sixty and sixty-five degrees. If a room is too cold (e.g., fifty-four degrees), dreams tend, for unknown reasons, to become unpleasant and highly emotional. On the other hand, if a room is too hot (e.g., seventy-five degrees), people wake up and move in bed more frequently. Dr. Kleitman found that sleep was more likely to be interrupted in the summer than in the winter.

Thus, overheating and overcooling your room will not only expend unnecessary energy but also disturb your sleep.

Unless you have a fetish for the exotic, any reasonably comfortable bed and mattress is fine for sleep. Although well-constructed mattresses may be necessary for those with specific orthopedic problems, they do not offer any advantage for the typical sleeper. Contrary to popular belief, curvature of the spine will not ensue from sleeping on a sagging mattress or in a curled-up position.

Whom you are or are not in bed with is more important than what you sleep on. Tensions between bedmates will interfere with falling asleep. One study of couples who were good sleepers revealed that they enjoyed more delta sleep when they slept apart than when they slept together. As Dr. Peter Hauri notes, "Sleeping together may be good for marital bliss, but sleeping apart does seem to deepen sleep by preventing disturbances when the partner changes position."

Capitalizing on people's zealous desire to sleep, the media perpetrate the myth that sleep can be purchased. Vibrating beds, water beds, "magic-motion" beds, earplugs, eyeshades, air purifiers, and contraptions emitting the sounds of raindrops are but a few of the paraphernalia marketed to tantalize the insomniac with visions of sleep. Although these devices may help some people sleep, I would caution you against indiscriminately opening your pocketbook to buy them. Sleep is not for sale.

Knowing the basic facts about sleep, you now will be able to complete the assessment in the following chapter and take advantage of the remedies offered throughout this book. And you can do all of this without a zillion expensive gadgets.

CHAPTER THREE

Assessing Your Sleep

You are about to embark on a pivotal step in overcoming insomnia. By assessing your sleep, you will not only learn a good deal about your sleep, but you will also learn how to obtain the maximum benefit from this book.

Your initial step in performing your assessment will be to determine if you have a sleep problem. Reaching this conclusion might seem like a straightforward proposition; either you sleep well or you don't. Unfortunately, it's not so simple. Without a polysomnograph, it is impossible to obtain an accurate measure of the quality and quantity of sleep. Furthermore, many insomniacs mistakenly, though unintentionally, exaggerate the severity of their sleep problems.

By contrasting self-reports with polysomnographic recordings, repeated studies have shown that in comparison to "good sleepers," self-styled "insomniacs" are more likely to (a) underestimate the duration of their sleep, (b) underestimate the number of their nocturnal awakenings, (c) overestimate the length of their sleep latencies, and (d) overestimate the time they spent awake after initially falling asleep.

Dr. Lawrence Monroe found that men who believed it took them over an hour to fall asleep actually did so in fifteen minutes. Dr. Dement showed that among patients who thought it took them more than an hour to drop off, almost 60 percent fell asleep within thirty minutes and 44 percent did so within fifteen minutes. These "insomniacs" slept forty-five minutes longer than they had estimated. Among patients who claimed to sleep less than five hours a night, only one in six was correct. Sixty-five percent of them snoozed for more than six hours. Thus, you probably are sleeping more than you believe.

If so, don't be embarrassed; unpleasant experiences, like not sleeping, seem to persist much longer than they actually do. When we are in severe pain, the agony often seems interminable. Moreover, if you are like many insomniacs, your sleep drifts between stages 0, 1, and 2. When this occurs, it feels as though you had been awake continuously, even though you slept most of the time. What is genuinely perceived as persistent sleeplessness is often light sleep punctuated by frequent mini-awakenings.

To aggravate matters, the self-labeled "insomniac" may dream about not sleeping. Phil, a Dartmouth College sophomore, bitterly complained of insomnia, claiming he was sleeping one hour a night. But his polysomnographic recordings revealed that he slept for a full eight hours a night. It was even more intriguing that when he was awakened from REM, Phil described struggling to fall asleep. His dreams of being unable to sleep were so vivid that he actually believed he was not sleeping. Once Phil learned that his sleep was normal, he was greatly relieved and thereafter slept like a log.

If, despite your best efforts, your own estimations of your sleep may be inaccurate, you might wonder why I will suggest you make such evaluations. Regardless of what the "truth" is or what the polysomnograph indicates, if you feel tired, you are tired. Although the machine is more precise in documenting sleeplessness than you are, your evaluation remains the most valid barometer of what you *experience*. After all, it is your experience, not the polysomnograph's, that counts.

Types of Insomnia

Insomnia has been defined as "a prolonged failure to procure sufficient sleep necessary to maintain health and well-being." Although an adequate definition, it lacks specificity. How long does a failure need to persist in order to be considered "prolonged?" What, specifically, is meant by "failure," "sufficient," "health," and "well-being"?

Just as definitions of insomnia have been controversial, so too have classifications of insomnia.* In general, however, there are four types of insomnia.

1. *Drug-induced Insomnia:* This problem occurs in those people who at least twice a week use hypnotics, alcohol, or other drugs in order to sleep.

2. *Sleep Disorders:* This group includes disruptions of sleep and wakefulness that follow a *specific* pattern but that are not caused by drugs or alcohol. These may be primarily disorders of sleep, such as narcolepsy, sleepwalking, or nightmares. They may also be disturbances of sleep secondary to medical diseases (e.g., asthma) or psychiatric conditions (e.g., depression).

3. *Biorhythm disturbances:* Your internal "biological clock," which is geared to a twenty-four-hour sleep-wake cycle, partially determines your pattern of sleep. This cycle, and therefore your sleep, can be disrupted by flying across time zones (jet lag), working irregular shifts, or following erratic day-night schedules.

4. *Nonspecific insomnia:* When there is no known cause for sleeplessness, it is called "nonspecific insomnia." Most types of insomnia fall into this residual category.

*The most recent official classification of sleep problems by the Sleep Disorders Classification Committee of the Association of Sleep Disorders Center is published in *Sleep 2*, no. 1 (1979):1–137. Although technically superior to the one listed here, the official classification is unnecessarily complex for our purposes.

If you are to obtain the maximum benefit from this book, you should first identify which of these four kinds of insomnia you have.

Self-Assessment

Numerous drugs, including alcohol, can affect not only your sleep, but your daytime alertness, as well. Indeed, if you are using *any* of the following substances within *two* hours of bedtime *more than twice* a week, you *may* have a drug-induced insomnia:

Hypnotics (e.g., Dalmane, barbiturates)
Sedatives (e.g., Valium, Librium)
Alcohol (e.g., wine, beer, whiskey)
Recreational drugs (e.g., marijuana, hashish)
Antidepressants (e.g., Tofranil, Elavil)
Antihistamines (e.g., Benadryl, PBZ)
Major tranquilizers (e.g., Thorazine, Mellaril)
Stimulants (e.g., amphetamines, "diet pills," cocaine)
Narcotics (e.g., morphine, Demerol)
Over-the-counter sleeping aids (e.g., Sominex, Nytol)

If you are taking any of these types of drugs, the best way to use this book is to complete this chapter and then to read (in order) Chapters 9, 4–8, and 10.

Because the sudden cessation of the use of hypnotics, sedatives, or alcohol can severely disturb your sleep and at times lead to withdrawal symptoms, *do not abruptly discontinue their use.* I would further recommend that you do not alter your current intake of any drugs or alcohol until you've read Chapter 9 and have consulted your physician.

Keep in mind that your taking a drug that influences sleep or wakefulness does not *necessarily* mean that you have a drug-induced insomnia. On the other hand, you *might* have one; if so, it's worth checking out. By reading Chapter 9 first, you can make this determination, and if you do have this problem, you will learn what to do about it. Furthermore, while you are using any of these drugs, you will be unable to take full advantage of the sleep-inducing techniques suggested in Chapters 4–8. Once you are off these drugs, however, you will be able to reap the optimal benefits from these methods.

To determine if you possibly have a sleep disorder, you should complete the self-assessment form in Table 3.1. The table asks seventeen questions; a positive response to *any* of them indicates that you *might* have a sleep disorder. In that case, you can derive the maximum help from this book by reading (in order) Chapters 10 and 4–9. Chapter 10 will help you confirm if you have a sleep disorder, and, if so, what you can do about it. If it turns out that you do have one, it's essential to remedy it *before* using the sleep-promoting techniques in Chapters 4–9. If you believe you have *both* a possible drug-induced insomnia *and* a possible sleep disorder, I'd suggest you read (in order) Chapters 9–10 and 4–8.

3.1 / SLEEP DISORDER SELF-ASSESSMENT FORM

Instructions: If you answer "yes" to any of the following questions, you *might* have a sleep disorder. If you so reply, pay special attention when reading Chapter 10, to the discussion of the sleep disorder(s) mentioned in the right-hand column of all those questions answered affirmatively.

NO.	QUESTION	YES	NO	POSSIBLE SLEEP DISORDER
1.	Do you, for no apparent reason, abruptly fall asleep or have an irresistible urge to sleep at inappropriate times?			Narcolepsy
2.	Do your muscles suddenly give out when you experience a strong emotion, such as when you laugh, cry, or become angry or tense?			Narcolepsy

NO.	QUESTION	YES	NO	POSSIBLE SLEEP DISORDER
3.	During the past two months, have you seen imaginary sights, or heard imaginary voices on falling asleep?			Narcolepsy
4.	During the past two months have you experienced a period of at least ten seconds, on awakening, during which you could not move?			Narcolepsy
5.	Do you snore *and* have trouble sleeping *or* feel constantly tired during the day?			Sleep apnea
6.	During the past month, have you awakened at night gasping for air?			Sleep apnea
7.	During the day, do you routinely experience an irrisistible urge to sleep, even though you slept sufficiently the previous night?			Hypersomnia, Narcolepsy, Sleep apnea
8.	In the past month, on falling asleep have your legs involuntarily twitched or kicked about every 20 to 40 seconds for more than two continuous minutes?			Kicking legs, (Nocturnal myoclonus)
9.	During the past month, have you had, at bedtime, a "crawling" or aching sensation in your legs which is alleviated by walking?			Restless legs
10.	Do you sleepwalk?			Sleepwalking
11.	During the past month, have you awakened from a frightening dream or in a state of panic?			Nightmares, Night terrors

Table continues on next page

NO.	QUESTION	YES	NO	POSSIBLE SLEEP DISORDER
12.	While asleep, do you grind your teeth for no apparent reason?			Tooth grinding (Bruxism)
13.	Have you felt *profoundly* depressed or hopeless for at least the past two weeks?			Major depression, Manic-depressive illness
14.	For at least the past two weeks, have you had *more than two* of the following: (a) poor appetite, (b) unintentional weight loss, (c) unrealistic feelings of guilt, (d) preoccupation with death or suicide, (e) difficulty concentration, (f) slowed or agitated movements, (g) markedly diminished sexual interest, or (h) an inability to experience pleasure or a pervasive loss of interest in people or activities that you previously enjoyed?			Major depression, Manic-depressive illness
15.	For at least the past seven days, have you had *more than one* of the following: (a) persistent uncalled-for elation, (b) hyperactivity, (c) grandiose schemes, (d) continual very rapid speech, (e) unreasonable spending sprees, or (f) persistent and uncalled-for irritability with people?			Manic depressive illness (also note the section on depression.)
16.	Do persistent, intrusive, "senseless," or "silly" thoughts prevent you from sleeping at least twice a week?			Obsessive-compulsive disorder

NO.	QUESTION	YES	NO	POSSIBLE SLEEP DISORDER
17.	Do you have heart disease, ulcers, asthma, thyroid problems, or epilepsy?			Heart disease, ulcers, asthma, hyperthyroidism, hypothyroidism, epilepsy (accordingly)

Except among shift workers, jet travelers, and those who follow highly erratic sleep-wake schedules, biorhythmic disturbances are relatively uncommon. Therefore, although the detection and alleviation of biorhythmic sleep problems are discussed in Chapter 8, it still would be preferable, if you have these difficulties, for you to read the preceding Chapters (4–7) beforehand.

If your sleeplessness does not fit into any of the first three categories, you probably have "nonspecific insomnia."* I say "probably," because many people incorrectly assume they have insomnia.

You have a genuine case of insomnia if you have had *sleeplessness and daytime fatigue lasting for at least a month*. If you have sleeplessness *without* daytime fatigue, you are merely an efficient, although brief, sleeper. Even if you have both sleeplessness and daytime fatigue, but if they have lasted for only a week or so, your plight, however, unsettling, hardly deserves to be called insomnia. After all, occasional sleeplessness is part of the human condition and readily disappears without active intervention. To decide if you have nonspecific insomnia, you should have a clear idea of what precisely is meant by "sleeplessness" and by "daytime fatigue."

You have sleeplessness if you suffer from any *one* of the following problems at least twice a week:

*Sleep experts often refer to "nonspecific insomnia" as "idiopathic insomnia," which is a fancy way of saying "insomnia due to unknown causes."

• Taking more than thirty minutes to fall asleep
• Waking up in the middle of the night and being unable
to fall back to sleep within thirty minutes
• Sleeping less than six and a half hours at night

Symptoms of daytime fatigue include loss of pep, tiredness,
and lethargy. These symptoms are only significant in terms
of evaluating insomnia if they are not due to physical
conditions, such as anemia, infections, or hypothyroidism
(underactive thyroid). If you have been chronically fatigued,
you should be examined by your physician in order to rule
out the existence of any underlying illness. Because everybody experiences some daytime fatigue regardless of how
much he or she sleeps, it is hard to distinguish normal from
problematic fatigue. As a rough guideline, however, you
can say you have significant daytime fatigue if it interferes
with your ability to function at least twice a week.

If you meet the above criteria for sleeplessness *and*
daytime fatigue, and if both symptoms have persisted for at
least a month, you have the dubious honor of qualifying for
nonspecific insomnia. In that case, the best way to employ
this book is to read it straight through (Chapters 4–10).

Using This Book

Having completed your self-assessment, you are ready to
overcome insomnia. Before doing so, however, check out
Figure 3.1 which summarizes the most effective and safest
route you should follow in using this program based on your
self-assessment.

As the Figure indicates, if you are principally concerned
about your child's sleep, rather than your own, I would
recommend that, though you should read the entire book,
you start with Chapter 11 and then proceed to Chapter 10.
If, after you implement the suggestions in these chapters,
your child still has difficulties, Chapters 4–9 will provide
you with some additional useful advice.

Monitoring Your Progress

Some people find it extremely helpful to monitor their progress *systematically*. Others find it a drag. There are, however, good reasons for doing so. If you maintain a daily-sleep log before you start using the remedies in this book, you might discover that your sleep is more erratic, or on the other hand, less severe, than you thought.

Once you actually begin employing this program, it is

FIGURE 3.1
HOW TO USE THIS BOOK

POSSIBLE DRUG-INDUCED INSOMNIA
Read Chapters 9, 4–8, and 10

POSSIBLE SLEEP DISORDER
Read Chapters 10 and 4–9

POSSIBLE DRUG-INDUCED INSOMNIA *and* POSSIBLE SLEEP DISORDER
Read Chapters 9, 10 and 4–8

NONSPECIFIC INSOMNIA *or* POSSIBLE BIORHYTHM DISTURBANCES
Read Chapters 4–10

CHILDHOOD SLEEP PROBLEMS
Read Chapters 11, 10, and 4–9

often gratifying to see your improvement documented in black and white. In addition to enjoying better sleep, recording your advances can be a valuable source of encouragement. Some of my patients have been so proud of their accomplishments with this program that they have constructed a chart illustrating their gains for the entire family to view. But even if you're less exhibitionistic, keeping such a chart for yourself alone can provide you some much-needed support.

Another, and possibly more important reason, is that a progress chart can show you which one of the many sleep-inducing techniques has assisted you the most. For example, in the next chapter you will see how changes in diet, exercise, and sleep schedules can all overcome insomnia. Let's say you adopted a soporific diet on the first day, started to exercise on the fourth day, and altered your sleep schedule on the seventh. By the end of the week you would have made three major changes in order to rid yourself of insomnia. Assuming your sleep improves, how do you know which technique—or combination of techniques—is doing the trick? If, by systematically monitoring your progress, you have discovered that your sleep *began* to improve on the fifth day, then it is clear that diet and exercise were the valuable remedies and that altering your sleep schedule was unnecessary. This method of evaluation is one of the ways a doctor figures out whether a particular treatment is helping a patient. You should be as critical and as scientific as a doctor. After all, it is vital for you to know which specific method works best for *you*. This information could be especially useful, if your sleep difficulties should recur. You would then know immediately which technique to employ, without having to repeat the entire program.

If you wish to monitor your progress, and I hope you do, I'd suggest using a procedure that offers you sufficient information without being so cumbersome that you'll eventually abandon it. Therefore, I'd recommend that you keep track of:

Sleep Latency—that is, the approximate number of minutes between when you go to bed and when you initially fall asleep.

Time Awake in the Middle of the Night—that is, the approximate number of minutes you were awake after you initially fell asleep, but before you finally got up in the morning.

Total Sleep Time—that is, the approximate number of hours you slept that night. Do not include time you napped during the day or the time you were awake in the middle of the night.

Fatigue Rating—that is, the *average* amount of fatigue you experience the *following* day. To calculate your fatigue ratings, use the following scale:*

1. Feeling active and vital; wide awake
2. Functioning at a high level, but not at peak; able to concentrate
3. Relaxed, awake, not at full alertness; responsive
4. A little foggy; not at peak; let down
5. Fogginess, beginning to lose interest in remaining awake; body feels slowed down
6. Sleepiness; prefer to be lying down; fighting sleep; woozy; hard to concentrate or thoughts slowed down
7. Almost in reverie; feel that you are about to fall asleep or that it is a struggle to stay awake
8. Asleep; napping

The more ratings you make throughout the day, the more accurate will be your score. Sleep researchers often have their clients perform hourly ratings all day long. Although such precision will yield more valid scores, many patients, in practice, become bored rating themselves so often and eventually forget to do it at all. I'd suggest a compromise: Make *three* ratings a day and *average* the results. If you conduct only one rating a day, it may not accurately reflect your fatigue for the entire day.

I would recommend that you perform these ratings at 10 A.M., 2 P.M., and 6 P.M. There's nothing special about these particular times. But whichever times you choose, try

*This scale derives from the Stanford Sleepiness Scale prepared by the Stanford University Medical Center's Sleep Disorders Center.

to space them evenly (e.g., four to five hours apart). Also make sure you use the same times from day to day. If you take your ratings at different times every day, biorhythmic fluctuations, as you will see in Chapter 8, will distort the validity of your determinations.

Sleep Methods Employed—that is, indicate which techniques you have used that day.

Table 3.2 presents a typical progress chart, taken from one of my patients. As you will note, there is a "baseline night"—that is, measurements showing how she slept *before* using any sleep-inducing method. In truth, this baseline night was the average of ten consecutive nightly baseline recordings. Because a single night's baseline assessment may be aberrant, one to two weeks of baseline measurements will more accurately reflect your typical sleep pattern. By comparing your baseline scores with those attained after you start the program, you will be able to determine if these sleep-inducing approaches have produced a substantial improvement.

In measuring how long you sleep, estimations will suffice. As I indicated earlier, exact measurements are not only difficult to obtain without a polysomnograph, but they also are apt to be inaccurate. Your ratings will give you a *general* idea of how you are sleeping. Staring at a clock in order to make more precise determinations will merely aggravate your insomnia. So stick with approximations; they'll adequately suit your purpose.

If you keep a progress chart, maintain it for as long as you use this program. By doing so, you'll be able to detect what's been helpful. From the patient's progress chart in Table 3.2, it became clear that the addition of exercise to her soporific diet accounted for her vastly improved sleep and fatigue scores. Additional evidence for this conclusion came from the entries for the final Wednesday and Thursday on her chart. On those days she continued to diet and to exercise, but she stopped taking tryptophan, a sleep-inducing substance. Because her greatly improved sleep persisted without tryptophan, diet and exercise turned out to be the critically effective remedies.

3.2 / TYPICAL PROGRESS CHART

NIGHT	SLEEP LATENCY	TIME AWAKE IN THE MIDDLE OF THE NIGHT	TOTAL SLEEP TIME	FATIGUE SCORE	SLEEP METHODS EMPLOYED		
					DIET	EXERCISE	TRYPTOPHAN
Baseline	90 min.	120 min.	3½ hrs.	6.6			
Tuesday 2/12/80	60 min.	80 min.	4½ hrs.	6.3	X		
Wednesday 2/13/80	60 min.	90 min.	5 hrs.	6.6	X		
Thursday 2/14/80	50 min.	75 min.	4½ hrs.	6.0	X		
Friday 2/15/80	20 min.	10 min.	5¾ hrs.	4.3	X	X	
Saturday 2/16/80	10 min.	—	6¼ hrs.	2.3	X	X	
Sunday 2/17/80	10 min.	—	6¼ hrs.	1.3	X	X	
Monday 2/18/80	10 min.	—	6¾ hrs.	1.3	X	X	X
Tuesday 2/19/80	10 min.	—	6½ hrs.	1.3	X	X	X
Wednesday 2/20/80	10 min.	—	7.0 hrs.	1.3	X	X	
Thursday 2/21/80	10 min.	—	7.0 hrs.	1.3	X	X	

Your progress chart should be completed daily. Once you skip a day, you'll be apt to neglect monitoring your sleep altogether. I'd also recommend that, except for the fatigue scores, you fill out the chart the very first thing in the morning. If you do so later in the day, you're likely to have greater difficulty remembering exactly how long you slept or were awake the preceding night.

Having made a commitment to this program, learned about sleep, and performed a self-assessment, you are now prepared to enter the most crucial phase of this program— overcoming insomnia. For the persistence you've shown up to this point, give yourself a pat on the back and get ready for a good night's sleep.

CHAPTER FOUR

Improving Sleep
Habits

If man is a creature of habit, then sleep is a creation of habit. Since we spend a third of our lives asleep, it is not surprising that so much imagination has gone into developing effective sleep habits. Like the rest of us, King Louis XIV enjoyed slipping into a freshly made bed. Unlike the rest of us, he made sure that a bed was always available by having 413 of them. But before you rush out to buy another 412 beds, recall that a deprived Benjamin Franklin made do with only 4. Always experimenting, he would at night go from bed to bed until he discovered one to his liking. Mrs. Franklin complained that she could never find him in the dark. Perhaps she required a compass? Charles Dickens did. Believing that magnetic currents would induce sleep if they surged through the body's midline, he used a compass to guarantee that his bed was aligned due north and south. Or consider Mark Twain's advice: ''If you can't sleep, try lying on the end of the bed—then you might drop off.'' If this proposal does not appeal to you, how about something more conventional? Sarah Bernhardt slept in a coffin.

Although your sleep habits are, I hope, less bizarre, you do have them—whether or not you are conscious of them. Every night you may close the blinds, open a window, or

prop your head against *two* pillows. These actions have
become so routine that you rarely, if ever, think about them.
Only when something interferes with them do you fully
appreciate their importance. If the window is stuck, you
miss the fresh air. If the blinds will not close, the light
annoys you. If forced to sleep on only one pillow, you feel
uncomfortable. Inevitably, you *choose* to practice certain
sleep habits, and it bothers you not to be able to indulge in
them.

As an insomniac, you have the task of cultivating
habits that maximize your chances for the best possible
sleep. Most of your habits will help; but a few may not.
You need to know which are useful and which are
counterproductive. You also need to know if you are
overlooking certain habits that, if adopted, would improve
your sleep.

This chapter presents the twelve habits that are most
conducive to sleep. Good sleepers can blissfully ignore
them and still sleep like a log. For you, however, these
habits should not be broken; they can make all the difference
between having or not having a refreshing night's sleep.

Unlike the weird sleep habits of Bernhardt, Dickens,
Franklin, and Louis XIV, the following twelve routines can
claim an effectiveness buttressed by scientific evidence.
Although most useful for overcoming moderate sleeplessness,
they can even alleviate severe insomnia. You add one
method at a time, and the more of these habits you eventually combine, the more likely it is that you will be able to sleep.

Apart from the habits proposed here, you undoubtedly
perform other bedtime rituals. You may routinely stack your
notebooks so that they're ready to be whisked away to
school the next morning. You might be uncomfortable
unless you've inspected the house to make sure all the lights
have been turned off. When you finally slip into bed, you
automatically make certain that your blanket covers all of
you, except for your right leg, which "must" dangle over
the bedside. Keep these habits; they expedite and are necessary for sleep—at least for you. Faced with the instability
and uncertainty of sleep, you can be greatly assisted by the

stability and certainty afforded by the use of regular sleep-related practices. In short, maintain your previously established habits, *unless* they conflict with the following suggestions.

Use the proposed routines *every* day. Start with one and apply it for two to three days. Then add a second for several days, and, if necessary, move on to a third, and so forth. Regardless of how many habits you're implementing, be consistent. Don't skip a day. If these practices don't immediately improve your sleep, don't abandon them. Be patient.

But how will you know if adopting certain habits is paying off? The best way to tell is by carefully and systematically recording your sleep and daytime fatigue ratings on a progress chart, like the one in Table 3.2. As Chapter 3 explained, if you compare your sleep and fatigue ratings with the habits you've employed, you can readily determine which of them are the most helpful.

So let's begin!

Habit 1—Reduce Excessive Noise

To "sleep soundly" is a contradiction. Sound disrupts sleep. If you are in a light stage of sleep, a loud noise, such as a sonic boom, can readily awaken you. Even if you are in REM sleep a sudden intense noise may arouse you, unless the sound is incorporated into your dream. For example, on a Fourth of July evening Carol's dream about a family reunion was abruptly terminated by exploding firecrackers. The same fireworks did not awaken her husband, because they became part of the "soundtrack" for his dream about a combat experience. If you are in deep (delta) sleep, noise may lighten your sleep to stage 2 or 1. Thus, a blaring trumpet can lighten and thereby disturb your sleep, even though you neither awake from it nor can recall it the following morning.

Try your best to attenuate loud noises. If you live near an airport or cacophonous traffic, you may wish to soundproof your bedroom. Soundproofing may be impractical or unnecessary, but using earplugs is not. Remember, even if you are not awakened by loud noises, the quality and the depth of your sleep may be disturbed by noise. By wearing earplugs, however, you may sleep longer and feel better the next day. Because they increase the number of nighttime awakenings and the amount of stage 1 sleep, episodic loud noises are especially detrimental to sleep. Therefore, by masking intermittent sounds, the constant noise of a fan or of an air conditioner can also substantially improve sleep.

The goal here is to reduce sound, not to eliminate it. Like air pollution, background noise is inescapable. Quixotic attempts to eradicate sound completely will fail, leading to more distress and more sleepless nights. By limiting your efforts to muffling loud noises, you not only will succeed, but will significantly improve the quality of your sleep. Don't worry about annoyances like dripping water faucets. Let them drip! Once you've established good sleeping habits, they will cease to bother you.

The disrupting effect of noise *during* sleep is clear; whether noise interferes with *falling* asleep is another matter. For most of you it is easier to drop off in a reasonably quiet room. On the other hand some people prefer, perhaps insist on, being lulled to sleep by music. Music can relax you; it can also distract you from obsessive thoughts whose intrusiveness prevents you from placing your mind, and therefore, your body at ease. Music, if it is to be used to sleep by, should neither stimulate nor irritate; it should calm. "Rock 'n' Roll to Sleep" will never be a hit. It is too arousing or too annoying to be soporific. Music should be pleasant, but unengaging. If *you* like falling to sleep with it, but your bedmate does not—music of any kind interferes with some people's sleep—purchase an inexpensive pillow-speaker or an earphone at any radio or TV shop.

Concerned about the erratic sleep habits of her husband Philip V of Spain, Elizabeth Farnese devised a scheme. This eighteenth-century king had a few quirks. Among these was an aversion to shaving and to having his bed linen changed. He was also reported to have worn the same clothes for a year and a half, even when asleep—which wasn't often.

Chronically unable to sleep, Philip was a mess. Because the reclusive monarch resented visitors, the queen tried to cheer him up by staging a recital in the chamber adjacent to the king's palace bedroom at La Granja near Segovia. For the occasion she hired the famous castrato Farinelli. According to Sir William Coxe, the British ambassador to the Spanish court, Philip was so enthralled by Farinelli's singing that after the completion of the second air he sent for the vocalist, lavished him with praise, and promised him anything he wanted. In exchange Farinelli, who by this time had become the première singer of Europe, sang the same four songs to Philip for five hours every night for ten years. Although the king never became a paragon of mental health, the monotonous repetition of Farinelli's sweet-floating music helped Philip sleep, so that he could more effectively attend to matters of state.

As a more practical alternative to hiring a singer to put you to sleep, you may wish to purchase a white-noise machine, which generates soothing sounds of rain, surf, or waterfalls. You can buy one for between twenty-two and ninety dollars. Its main purpose is to camouflage disturbing background noise and thus to make it easier to fall asleep. It is hard to say whether such devices accomplish this objective, because of random noise, the few subjects who have been observed fell asleep on the average nine minutes sooner with the machine than without it. Whether nine additional minutes of sleep is worth the money is up to you. Remember, boring background music or a humming fan may have the same effect, both are certainly less expensive.

Although some prefer rainfalls and others music, for most people the "hush of night" will be most conducive to sleep. Creating a relatively quiet environment is undoubtedly the first good sleep habit to cultivate.

Habit 2—Maintain a Moderate Room Temperature

As Chapter 2 pointed out, excessive heat or cold interferes with obtaining optimal sleep. The old wives' tale that cold air improves sleep is quaint but wrong. Old wives aside, your bedroom should be of moderate temperature—that is, between sixty and sixty-five degrees Fahrenheit (or about sixteen and eighteen degrees centigrade). But since individual preferences vary considerably, it is most important for you to select a room temperature that affords you maximum comfort.

Habit 3—Exercise for Sleep

If used judiciously, consistent exercise will extend and deepen sleep. Before joining a herd of joggers, however, exercise a little caution.

Studies show that athletes have more delta sleep than nonathletes. But when athletes fail to get their customary exercise, they have less deep sleep that night. Unfortunately, the converse does not hold. Exercising frantically on a given day does not deepen the nonathlete's sleep that night. Moreover, the ensuing aches and pains may keep you awake. Those findings for athletes also apply to people who stay in good physical condition. Therefore, a reasonable amount of *daily* exercise promotes sleep.

To enjoy the maximum soporific effect, you should exercise in the afternoon or early evening. Morning exercise occurs too early to influence sleep. Exercise immediately before bedtime will arouse and stimulate, making it harder to fall asleep.

The two major obstacles to using exercise for sleep are laziness and overzealousness. Writing to Thomas Randolph in 1786, Thomas Jefferson prescribed that "not less than two hours a day should be devoted to exercise." Referring to that letter, John Kennedy observed, "If the man who wrote the Declaration of Independence, was secretary of state, and twice president, could give it [exercise] two hours, our children can give it ten or fifteen minutes." So too can adults. Unless you are immobilized by a plague or stuffed in a strait jacket, there is no earthly reason for you to avoid participating in a moderate exercise program.

Try walking to your job. If you prefer, retrieve the old bike and pedal to work. Walk up a few flights of stairs instead of riding the elevator. The opportunities for exercise are plentiful, and with a little imagination and a little more determination you can readily incorporate it into your daily routine. It may also be fun.

Exercise is beneficial when moderate, but dangerous when sudden or excessive. The zealousness, akin to a religious conversion, with which some people discover salvation in jogging, running, and other frenetic activities inspired Chauncey Depew to observe, "I get my exercise acting as pallbearer to my friends who exercise." If you are unaccustomed to daily exercise, begin slowly and every day increase your activity a little. Superb exercise programs can be found in Dr. John Farquhar's paperback *The American Way of Life Need Not Be Hazardous to Your Health* (New York: Norton, 1978) or in Dr. Kenneth Cooper's *The New Aerobics* (New York: Bantam Books, 1970).

If you have diabetes, arthritis, high blood pressure, or heart disease, check with your physician before launching any exercise program. Moderate exercise is healthy; physical machismo is stupid.

Habit 4—Have Sex for Sleep

To speak of sex as a sleep habit may seem odd to some and wishful thinking to others. It might also seem contradictory to state that exercise at bedtime prevents sleep, while sex at bedtime facilitates sleep. Nevertheless, gratifying sex is an excellent soporific.

Whereas satisfying sex leads to satisfying sleep, sex that is physically uncomfortable or emotionally distressing can aggravate insomnia. If sexual problems interfere with your sleep, it is valuable to discuss these matters honestly yet sensitively with your partner. By doing so, you will not only obtain a better night's sleep but also enrich your relationship.

Although we are said to live in a sexually permissive society, many of us experience considerable difficulties in discussing sexual problems openly and lovingly. The tyranny of Victorian morality has been superceded by the tyranny of sexual liberation. Today men and women often feel guilty and ashamed if they are anything less than sexual superstars. Being preoccupied with proving their sexual prowess, they are unable simply to enjoy lovemaking. Sex therapists refer to this phenomenon as "performance anxiety," and it often renders sex unsatisfying and sleep unobtainable. Nagging questions—"How well did I perform?"; "Will he (or she) think I reached orgasm?"; "Did I climax too quickly?" —are bound to keep you awake. Whether sex will enhance or inhibit sleep thus depends on whether it occurs in the context of a supportive, trusting, and loving relationship.

If you are without a sexual partner, masturbation is an equally effective soporific. This readily available, potentially pleasurable activity is still enshrouded in ignorance, guilt, and superstition. In a Graham Greene short story an old man dying in a hospital cancer ward reflects on his life and concludes that masturbation *did* lead to cancer. But what Greene spoofs others scorn. If the idea of masturbation offends you, then masturbation will not help you sleep. On the other hand, if it is emotionally and morally acceptable to you, it will facilitate sleep.

Habit 5—Eliminate Evening Caffeine

At the turn of this century an English physician described the typical coffee drinker as a person who was "tremulous, loses his self-command, is subject to fits of agitation and depression, and has a haggard appearance. . . . a renewed dose of the poison gives temporary relief, but at the cost of future misery." Today we merely say that he suffers from "coffee nerves."

Americans consume 400 million cups of coffee a day, which comes to at least two billion pounds of coffee a year. A boss who does not permit a coffee break is viewed by his employees as inflicting cruel and unusual punishment. Chances are, therefore, that you'll be less than ecstatic when I suggest you drink no coffee within six hours of bedtime.

Although coffee is widely recognized as a stimulant which disrupts sleep, the prevalence of caffeine in other beverages and in medications is not so fully appreciated. Table 4.1 lists the common sources and the amounts of

4.1 / COMMON SOURCES OF CAFFEINE*

SOURCE	AMOUNT OF CAFFEINE (IN MGS.)
Beverages	
Brewed coffee	100–150 per cup
Instant coffee	80–99 per cup
Tea	60–75 per cup
Decaffeinated coffee	2–4 per cup
Cola drinks	40–60 per glass
Prescription Medications	
Cafergot	100 per tablet
Darvon compound	32 per capsule
Fiorinal	40 per tablet
Migral	50 per tablet
Over-the-Counter Pain Relievers	
Anacin, aspirin compound, Bromo-Seltzer, Cope, Easy-Mens, Empirin compound, Midol, Vanquish	32 per tablet
Excedrin	60 per tablet
Pre-Mens	66 per tablet
Many Over-the-Counter Cold Pills	30 per capsule
Many Over-the-Counter Stimulants	100 per tablet

*This table is a slightly modified version of one presented by Dr. John F. Greden in "Anxiety or Caffeinism: A Diagnostic Dilemma," *American Journal of Psychiatry 131* (1974): 1090.

caffeine`in them. Review the table carefully. Since caffeine
is so ubiquitous, you are probably underestimating your
total caffeine consumption.

Although there are wide variations for different individuals, more than 250 milligrams of caffeine can prolong sleep
latency, diminish delta sleep, and increase the number of
nighttime awakenings. Nervousness, irritability, agitation,
headache, rapid heart rate, tremulousness, and occasional
muscle twitches can also result from the intake of more than
250 milligrams of caffeine. As if all this weren't enough,
some heavy coffee drinkers experience a ''pins-and-needles''
sensation on their body, ringing in their ears, and visual
flashes before their eyes. All of these symptoms are especially pronounced among middle-aged and elderly caffeine
users.

The stimulating effects of caffeine peak between two and
four hours, linger for seven hours, and may persist for as
long as twenty hours following ingestion. Consequently,
caffeine may be disrupting your sleep long after you believe
its influence has worn off.

Ideally, caffeine—not just coffee, but *all* caffeine—should
not be consumed within six hours of bedtime. If this seems
unnecessarily harsh, remember that the stimulant effects of
caffeine are greater and persist longer than you imagine. By
abstaining from caffeine you will fall asleep sooner and have
a more refreshing night's sleep. In addition, once you're
sleeping better, your ''need'' for morning coffee will diminish.

But if you are an insatiable caffeine consumer, do not
stop abruptly. Chances are you won't stick to sudden
abstinence. Instead, reduce your caffeine intake to no more
than 250 milligrams within six hours of bedtime. Maintain
this moderate regimen for two weeks. Subsequently, taper
your caffeine use by roughly ten percent a night. In this
manner it will be easier to refrain from coffee, tea, and cola
over the long haul—and that's what counts.

Habit 6—Stop Smoking

Although having an occasional cigarette may be relaxing, smoking heavily causes insomnia. Three-pack-a-day smokers take longer to fall asleep, awake more frequently, and have less REM and stage 4 sleep. Because nicotine withdrawal initially appears two to three hours after the last puff, heavy smokers often arise from their sleep craving yet another cigarette.

Within three days of giving up tobacco, however, the heavy smoker's sleep improves dramatically. Almost immediately he drops off more quickly and sleeps without interruption. After two weeks REM and stage 4 sleep return to normal.

Unlike the heavy smoker, the light smoker does not find his sleep stages significantly altered by his habit. But the typical one-pack-a-day smoker does stay awake at night an average of nineteen minutes more than does the nonsmoker, mainly because it takes the former fourteen minutes longer to fall asleep. When the relatively light smoker abruptly abstains from nicotine, his time spent awake and his sleep latency decrease within three days by 45 percent and 65 percent, respectively. As a result, the former smoker now sleeps better.

There are several useful books and programs that can assist you in kicking the habit. Among the former is Dr. John Farquhar's paperback *The American Way of Life Need Not Be Hazardous to Your Health* (New York: Norton, 1978). He outlines a program which is similar to the one used by Smokenders, the nation's largest and possibly most successful antismoking organization. Smokenders claim that 92 percent of their graduates quit smoking initially and that a year later 70 percent have kept it up. It may be, as some independent investigators have maintained, that only 30 percent of participants still refrain from smoking after a year of the program. But if you don't start to quit, there's no way you will continue to quit.

The Smokenders course consists of eight two-hour ses-

sions, conducted weekly by one of its graduates. Terry
Hughes from Smokenders describes the program: "For the
first five weeks, you continue to smoke as you are getting
prepared to quit without climbing the walls. 'Cut-off' day
arrives after the fifth meeting. You return for three meetings
after 'cut-off' to help you cope with your new nonsmoking
life."

In 1981 the fee for the program was $345. It's costly, but,
in terms of your life, so is smoking. If you want further
information, write to Smokenders, 37 North Third Street,
Easton, PA 18042, or call their world headquarters toll-free
at 1–800–227–2334.

Cigarette smoking disrupts sleep because large amounts
of nicotine are inhaled. Because it does not involve inhaling, the use of a pipe, cigars, or snuff will not substantially
affect your sleep.

Habit 7—Avoid Nightcaps

Having an alcoholic beverage before bedtime is a time-
honored but not a time-tested tradition. Clearly, a glass of
wine or a can of beer will get you to sleep faster. Once you
are asleep, however, this innocent nightcap fragments sleep;
REM and delta sleep are suppressed and fluctuations between sleep stages are accelerated. The effect of alcohol on
sleep is thus deceptive. Although the insomniac knows that
a drink facilitates getting to sleep, he is unaware that it
prevents refreshing sleep. Feeling unrested, he naturally, but
mistakenly, assumes that alcohol is a solution to and not the
cause of his sleep problem.

Many alcoholics are former insomniacs who drank themselves to sleep. Alcoholism is discussed in greater detail in
Chapter 9; at this point remember that alcohol interferes
with the sleep of even the most temperate of souls. You
don't have to be pie-eyed for alcohol to disrupt your sleep.
Alcohol not only causes direct physiological distortions of
normal sleep patterns; it is also a strong enough diuretic to

awaken you several times a night to go to the bathroom. Let the drink you have with dinner, therefore, be the last one for the evening.

Habit 8—Nibble Your Way to Sleep

The great British physician Sir William Gull wrote, "I do not know what a brain is, and I do not know what sleep is, but I do know that a well-fed brain sleeps well." Twentieth-century research has substantiated this nineteenth-century speculation. It has been found that whereas those who are gaining weight sleep more, those who are shedding pounds sleep less. People who follow semistarvation diets often experience sleeplessness. In a zealously weight-conscious society, it is probable that crash dieting is a major, though widely unrecognized, cause of insomnia. When the dieter resumes eating normally, he also returns to sleeping normally.

It has been shown that grabbing a light snack before bedtime improves sleep. Make sure, however, that it is only a snack and not a feast. Digesting a large meal stimulates the body, lightens sleep, and arouses the sleeper. On the other hand, small snacks, such as a glass of milk and a cookie, will help you doze off.

Speaking of food, you may be unusually sensitive to monosodium glutamate (MSG). Used as a flavor enhancer, MSG may cause symptoms akin to "coffee nerves," including insomnia. So if you're having trouble sleeping, avoid MSG. Because Chinese food often swims in MSG, the next time you go out for chop suey, specifically ask that it be prepared without MSG.

Habit 9—Take Tryptophan

As a child were you told that a cup of warm milk would put you to sleep? Do you feel tired after devouring a large steak? What do a steak and milk have in common so that they would both induce sleep? True, they both come from cows; but the real answer is that they both contain tryptophan (or 1-tryptophan), a naturally occurring amino acid. (Amino acids are the building blocks that make up proteins.) After tryptophan is digested, it travels via the blood stream to the brain, where it is converted into serotonin, or "sleep juice." Foods rich in tryptophan, such as meat, poultry, soybeans, and dairy products, are thus soporific.

When choosing a nighttime snack, pick one that is loaded with tryptophan. One or two cups of warm milk, Ovaltine, or Horlicks (a Scotch malted milk drink) contain sufficient tryptophan to lull you to sleep. If drunk about twenty minutes before bedtime, each of them makes a superb sleep-inducing snack.

Although Dr. Kleitman had recognized as early as 1937 the soporific influence of tryptophan-containing drinks, not until 1964 did Dr. Ernest Hartmann seriously experiment with tryptophan as a "sleeping pill." It is possible that within the next ten years tryptophan tablets may substantially obviate the need for conventional hypnotics. Unlike hypnotics, soporific doses of one to five grams of tryptophan are not habituating, do not alter normal physiological sleep, are free of side effects, and cannot give rise to allergic reactions. As Dr. Hartmann points out, "L-tryptophan should be one of the safer drugs available, since one to two grams are ingested daily in the normal diet."

In carefully performed studies Dr. Hartmann and others have shown that tryptophan significantly reduces sleep latency. When patients take tryptophan, they become tired but seldom feel "knocked out."

So far the Food and Drug Administration has not sanctioned the use of tryptophan as a sleeping pill. (But it is sold as a dietary supplement.) Its caution is understandable; all too often drugs that initially seem harmless turn out on long-term use to cause serious complications. As of now the long-range effects of tryptophan have not been sufficiently investigated. Nevertheless, since it is a naturally occurring substance, it is unlikely that any adverse consequences will be found.

Until further research has been completed, common sense dictates that the nightly use of tryptophan tablets should be avoided. But the occasional use of tryptophan pills and the nightly use of tryptophan-rich beverages are safe and effective ways to fall asleep.

Tryptophan tablets can be found in any health-food store and in the vitamins and minerals section of most pharmacies. Tryptophan is usually marketed as either 100-milligram or 500-milligram tablets. Though all available evidence suggests that 2,000 to 3,000 milligrams can be safely used at bedtime, Dr. Hartmann recommends taking 1,000 milligrams (one gram) of tryptophan about twenty minutes before retiring.

Prices for thirty, 500-milligram tablets usually range from $6.95 to $9.95; which is to say, a typical 1,000-milligram nightly dose costs between $.46 and $.66. Before you purchase tryptophan, make sure you do some comparative shopping. Although they have larger stocks of tryptophan, health-food centers are often more expensive than neighborhood pharmacies.

Habit 10—Establish a Regular Sleep Schedule

Each of us is biologically endowed with a sleep-wake cycle. One person's biological clock might be set for seven hours of sleep and seventeen hours of wakefulness. Another person's clock might establish a daily pattern of eight hours of sleep and sixteen of wakefulness. Your biological clock also plays a significant role in determining *when* you'll be awake and asleep. Under natural conditions you would get up and retire at roughly the same time every day.

But the exigencies of modern life often interfere with your normal sleep-wake cycle. Flying across time zones gives rise to jet lag. Staying up late on Saturday night or sleeping late the following morning disrupts your natural biorhythm. Of course, a life that conforms totally to the dictates of a biological clock is a boring life. Nevertheless, disruptions of biorhythms can give rise to insomnia. To overcome sleeplessness, you must reestablish your innate sleep-wake cycle.

Conversely, insomnia throws your biological clock out of gear. If you can't sleep at night, you're likely to nap during the day. But if you snooze in the afternoon, you'll have more difficulty falling asleep at night. Convinced that you're getting insufficient sleep, you might be tempted to turn in early. Once this pattern of napping and going to bed early becomes established, it upsets your entire sleep-wake cycle.

A common problem arising from this disturbance of the natural sleep-wake cycle is what Dr. Wilse Webb calls "Sunday-night insomnia." Why, out of all the nights of the week, should it be most difficult to fall asleep on Sunday night? As I explained in Chapter 2, the longer you are awake prior to bedtime, the faster you will fall asleep. In other words, as prior wakefulness expands, sleep latency contracts. Conversely, a short period of prior wakefulness lengthens the time it takes to fall asleep. This abbreviated prior wakefulness is the cause of Sunday-night insomnia. By sleeping late into Sunday morning and retiring early on Sunday night (in order to be refreshed for work on Monday), prior wakefulness is reduced at both ends. Consequently, it takes longer to drift off on Sunday than on any other night of the week.

If you are a normally good sleeper who wishes to overcome Sunday-night insomnia, just increase the number of hours you are awake before going to bed. By arising earlier, or by going to bed later, or both, you can expand your prior wakefulness. A longer interval of prior wakefulness also increases delta sleep and slightly prolongs nighttime sleep. Thus, by lengthening prior wakefulness, you will fall asleep faster and awake more refreshed.

The concept of prior wakefulness can be applied anytime you wish to get a better night's sleep on a particular occasion. Let's say you're an actress who has an important audition on Thursday, and you're concerned that the "jitters" will prevent you from sleeping on Wednesday night. To insure a refreshing Wednesday night sleep, you should get up several hours earlier on Wednesday morning.

Another way to guarantee a good night's sleep is to avoid all daytime naps. Naps reduce prior wakefulness. If you awake at 8 A.M. and retire at 11 P.M., you are awake for fifteen hours prior to bedtime. But if you nap from 1 P.M. to 3 P.M., for example, your prior wakefulness is reduced to eight hours. As a result, it takes you longer to fall asleep, you obtain less delta sleep, and you shorten your total nighttime sleep.

You can overcome insomnia by altering your sleep schedule in three ways:

1. *Do not nap.* Although many people can nap and still sleep normally at night, you, as an insomniac, are not one of them.

2. *Go to bed only when you're sleepy.* Don't retire at 11 P.M. just because you "always go to bed at 11 P.M." Unless you're sleepy, you'll merely lie awake worrying about why you can't sleep. The longer you fret, the longer it will take you to sleep.

You might ask, "If I don't go to bed until I'm sleepy, how will I ever get enough rest?" Don't worry, you will. Trust your body; it knows and will let you know when it needs to sleep. When the body's ready to sleep, it sleeps; if not, it won't. Going to bed only when you are sleepy is necessary if you are to restore a normal sleep-wake cycle.

3. *Arise at the same time every morning.* I cannot overemphasize this rule. Because it is much easier to force yourself to wake up than to sleep, the most effective way to maintain a regular sleep-wake cycle is to make sure that you get up at the same time every day. After several weeks, you'll even discover that a natural consequence of arising at the identical time is that you'll fall asleep at a regular hour.

During the week, this rule is easy to follow. Most people have to work at the same time every morning. On weekends, however, the normal tendency is to catch some extra shut-eye. But when you get additional sleep on the weekend, your natural sleep-wake cycle is disrupted.

By waking at the same time every morning, avoiding naps, and going to bed only when you are sleepy, your body can reestablish its normal biorhythmic sleep pattern. You also can readily determine your daily sleep requirement. If you routinely awake refreshed at 8 A.M. and become sleepy at 11 P.M., then you need nine hours of sleep (i.e., from 11 P.M. to 8 A.M.) If you constantly change the time you arise, it becomes harder to make this calculation.

By altering your sleep schedule in these three ways, you will reestablish your sleep-wake cycle, but not overnight. After your cycle has been out of kilter for a long time, it takes several weeks for it to return to normal. But the wait and transitory inconvenience are worth it. Once your sleep occurs in concert with your biological rhythm, it will improve.

Don't worry—you won't have to follow these rigid rules forever. As soon as your insomnia has been vanquished, you can vary, within reason, the time at which you arise in the morning.

Habit 11—Relax before Bedtime

Whoever first suggested counting sheep never had insomnia. If he had, he quickly would have discovered that he was more awake than before. Instead of relaxing you, counting sheep forces you to concentrate. Any prebedtime activity that stimulates the mind is bound to keep you awake. If you know in advance that you'll have to worry about a particular problem or to settle a difficult issue that night, do so at least an hour before retiring. Cramming for an exam, balancing the check book, or squabbling with your spouse is hardly conducive to sleep. If your mind is at rest, your body will follow suit.

Although the following chapter will describe a specific method for relaxing, there are many other simpler ways of calmly and serenely going to bed. Relaxing in a warm bath, reading a pleasant book, praying, or meditating will hasten sleep. Doing nothing but listening to peaceful music at the end of a hard day is a superb way to unwind. But whatever relaxes you, if you purposely set aside fifteen minutes before retiring to do it, falling asleep becomes easier.

Habit 12—Use Beds Only for Sleeping (Stimulus Control)

The sight of a bed can resurrect numerous memories and emotions. When you were a "bad girl," you were sent "straight to bed." You were born and will die in bed. You make love in bed, play in bed, and cry in bed. Given that you've spent a third of your life in bed, reflect for a moment on all that has happened in your bed. A bed is not merely another piece of furniture; it is a reminder of many of the milestones and key events of your life. If you are an insomniac, the very thought of your bed, and especially of trying to fall asleep in it, may provoke other, often disturbing feelings.

After insomnia becomes entrenched, the mere idea of going to bed may fill you with dread. As Dee, a thirty-seven-year-old patient of mine said, "As soon as the nightly TV news is over, I stare at my bed and shiver. I become tense at the very thought of spending another long night in that bed. My head throbs, my mouth becomes dry, I can hardly swallow. I know it's silly, but it's like my bed is an enemy whose sole mission is to prevent me from sleeping." She paused and then laughed. "How would you feel about sleeping on top of your enemy?"

For insomniacs like Dee the bed is not a comfortable haven, but an unavoidable adversary. Even if you are unaware of it, you may have become so conditioned that as the time to fall asleep approaches, you automatically view the bed with apprehension.

Because this feeling is so pervasive, behavioral psychologist Dr. Richard Bootzin successfully devised a *stimulus control* technique to induce sleep. The purpose of Bootzin's method is to get the insomniac to disassociate the sight of his bed from all unsettling and stimulating thoughts, and to get him to reassociate it with the ability to sleep. Consequently, apart from sex, you should use the bed for *nothing* but sleep. More specifically, at bedtime you should follow these five rules:

1. Go to bed only when you are sleepy.
2. Except for having sex and sleeping, do not read, listen to the radio or stereo, watch television, or do anything else in the bedroom, especially in bed. Throughout the day use the bedroom only for activities that cannot be performed elsewhere. Obviously, because it's impractical (if not bizarre) to dress in the kitchen, go ahead and do so in your bedroom. But otherwise, except for sleep and sex, avoid your bedroom.
3. If you're unable to fall asleep in roughly fifteen minutes, go into another room and do something relaxing. Fifteen minutes is merely a guideline. By staring at the clock or by counting minutes, you'll simply exacerbate the problems you have in falling asleep. So just give yourself enough, but not too much, time to drop off before you leave your bed.
4. When, and only when, you feel sleepy, return to bed.
5. If you still cannot fall asleep in about fifteen minutes— or at least when it's clear that you're not going to drift asleep promptly on this go-around—repeat steps 3 and 4 until you drop off.

After a year of insomnia, Dee tried this method. In two weeks her sleep returned to normal.

It was crucial for Dee, as it will be for you, to know in advance that this technique may entail three to six relatively sleepless nights before it restores your natural sleep-wake cycle. During the first several nights you may have to remain in another room for several hours before you feel sleepy. You may go to bed and get up again four to ten times during the night. Dee slept only two hours during each of the first four nights she employed this method. By the fifth night, however, she was out of her bedroom for a mere forty-five minutes. Although she felt slightly more fatigued during these initial days, she wisely resisted the temptation to nap. Over the ensuing nine days, by sticking assiduously to this plan, she gradually reduced the number of times she had to get up. By the fourteenth day, and thereafter, she fell asleep in ten minutes and slept through the night.

Once Dee realized that she actually had the power to overcome her dread of the bed and of going to sleep, she slept like a dream. A month later she remarked, "It's nice to see that your enemy can become your ally."

You may become antsy sitting around in another room waiting to feel sleepy. After all, what do you do to pass the time? It's the middle of the night and there is nobody to call. You can't go to a movie, and even the television has turned in for the evening. Most distressing is the perpetual thought that you will not get enough sleep. Instead of worrying about these matters, however, seize the opportunity to use these additional hours to catch up on all those unread newspapers, magazines, and books. Play solitaire. Listen to music. Read the Bible. Plan the meals for the week. Water the plants. Fix the bicycle you're going to exercise with. Do a crossword puzzle. Peruse an almanac; it's filled with delightful tidbits. Don't fuss about the time you *think* you have lost from sleep. Consider the extra time you now have available to enjoy yourself.

To employ stimulus control requires patience and willpower. If you have been conditioned for an extended period to dread going to bed, it may take three to six weeks for this method to improve your sleep. Though some people obtain substantial relief in four or five days, all too many insomniacs prematurely abandon this technique after several nights. The method is effective, but you must stick to it. Your spouse can be extremely helpful, especially during the first and most difficult week, by constantly encouraging you to adhere to this stimulus-control approach. Although sheer persistence and willpower on your part will make stimulus control work for you, there's nothing wrong with asking for some additional support. Moreover, don't worry about how long the method needs to be used in order to succeed. Just take one night at a time. Recognize and learn to appreciate that for every single night you keep to the program, you'll come a little closer to vanquishing insomnia.

Even after you have overcome insomnia, continue to use the bed only for sleep and sex. When an occasional sleepless night reappears—as happens to everyone—reapply Bootzin's method. By doing so, you will quickly recapture normal sleep before persistent insomnia can once again become entrenched.

Now you have a dozen scientifically proven methods for improving your sleep. For your convenience, they're summarized below.

SUMMARY OF SLEEP HABITS

1. Reduce excessive noise; wear earplugs if necessary.
2. Keep the room temperature between sixty and sixty-five degrees.
3. Exercise during the afternoon or early evening.
4. Engage in sexual activity, but only if satisfying.
5. Refrain from caffeine within six hours of sleep.
6. Abstain from cigarettes.
7. Do not drink alcoholic beverages after dinner.
8. Have a light snack before retiring. Avoid MSG.
9. Drink a cup of warm milk, Ovaltine, or Horlicks just before going to bed. Or try one gram of tryptophan about twenty minutes before bedtime.
10. Awake at the same time every day and go to bed only when you're sleepy. Avoid naps.
11. Avoid stimulating or intense mental activity during the hour before you go to sleep. Immediately before retiring, set aside fifteen minutes for some quiet relaxation.
12. Do not remain in bed for longer than fifteen minutes unless you are asleep or having sex. If you cannot fall asleep in fifteen minutes, leave the bedroom, try to relax, and return to bed only when you're sleepy.

But instead of applying them all at once, I'd suggest you begin by implementing a single habit for several days. With the exception of altering your sleep schedule and employing

Bootzin's stimulus control method (which both require one to six weeks to become fully effective), the sleep habits outlined in this chapter can work in two or three days. After using the first technique, add, if necessary, a second for a couple of days, and then a third, and so forth. By keeping your daily progress chart (Table 3.2), you can detect which of these methods is particularly helpful to you. If you start by practicing all of these habits at once, you will be unable to pinpoint those specific remedies that are responsible for your good night's sleep.

Eventually, you may use all twelve approaches together. The cumulative effects of these methods will clearly afford you the best possible chance of eliminating those long sleepless nights.

Knowing these habits is one thing; cultivating them is another. Make sure to practice them *every* day. Consistency and patience will pay off. Don't be slipshod. After all, you deserve nothing but the best.

CHAPTER FIVE

Relaxing to Sleep

If you're a tangle of nerves, you can't sleep. This chapter shows you how to untangle those nerves by relaxation.

When unable to sleep, you may be pestered by thoughts that plague your mind and tense your muscles. By learning progressive relaxation, however, you can rid yourself of these worries and tensions. As a result, you will be able to promptly drift asleep.

Nighttime Worries and Muscle Tension

Though everyone has worries, some can set them aside when they go to bed. Others "sleep on their problems"; they end up neither solving their problems nor sleeping. For many of us, our greatest worries surface at bedtime, when we are removed from the distractions of daily life. Lying in bed, we'll fret about everything that has gone awry during the day. Moreover, the very thought of sleep may provoke additional concerns.

Sleep has long been associated with death. Shelley wrote of "Death and his brother Sleep"; Shakespeare viewed sleep as "death's counterfeit." Historically, natives of Burma and of the Fiji Islands believed that the soul left the body on falling asleep and returned at daybreak. If a sleeper was awakened too early, his soul would be unable to reinhabit his body. Since a body without a soul was considered dead, prematurely waking someone was tantamount to murdering him. This tribal link between sleep and death persists in our bedtime prayers:

> Now I lay me down to sleep;
> I pray the Lord my soul to keep.
> If I should die before I wake,
> I pray the Lord my soul to take.

Sleep and death are linked not only in literature, folklore, and religion, but also in medicine. Many people die while asleep or in a coma, which appears as sleep.

Because sleep is a time of maximum vulnerability and minimum control, the thought of sleep conjures up other fears. Horror films exploit this theme. At nightfall thirsty vampires attack slumbering maidens, while innocent sleepers turn into werewolves. Television news, often watched just before retiring, reinforces our fears of being robbed, raped, or murdered while asleep.

Although hopefully your evening worries are less terrifying, you may still find something to fret about. It may be a family squabble or a mortgage payment. It may be an arthritic back or a union negotiation. At other times trivia may preoccupy you: "What should I wear tomorrow?" "What was the name of that song?" "Whom did my third cousin Isaac marry?" If nothing else, you'll worry about insomnia.

To fall asleep quickly, you must be able to rid your mind of these distractions. But very often the harder you try to divest yourself of intrusive thoughts, the more entrenched they become. What you need is a method that simultaneously unclutters your mind and promotes sleep.

While these worries are tying your mind into knots, they may be tying your skeletal muscles into knots. Skeletal muscles are those under voluntary control (e.g., face, arm, chest, stomach, and leg muscles). The tenser these muscles, the harder it is to relax, and therefore to sleep. If your muscles are tight and you want to sleep, you, and not your worries, must control your muscular tension.

Worries and muscular tension generate a vicious circle; the more the one increases, the more the other increases. By applying a relaxation technique, you can readily break that circle and pleasantly fall asleep. As many studies have repeatedly demonstrated, the progressive relaxation method advanced in this chapter hastens the onset of sleep by an average of 43 percent. Insomniacs using this technique also awake less frequently in the middle of the night and feel more refreshed in the morning.

Understanding Relaxation

Relaxation means different things to different people. Relaxing usually connotes playing golf, watching television, or puttering around the house. But in this chapter relaxation refers to the technique pioneered by Dr. Edmund Jacobson.

Dr. Jacobson has spent most of this century analyzing, developing, and refining his technique. He and his followers have successfully used relaxation methods in the treatment of insomnia, as well as of anxiety, obesity, heart diseases, high blood pressure, indigestion, ulcers, colitis, phobias, and many other conditions. Over the years Dr. Jacobson's basic technique has been modified depending on the disorder being healed and the predilections of the healer. There are many variations of his fundamental method; this book presents one that is especially conducive to sleep.

To obtain the maximum benefit from relaxation, you should know a little about how skeletal muscles function. Each muscle comprises many smaller muscle fibers, which are attached to minuscule nerve branches. When you want to flex a muscle, your brain speeds electrical impulses to the ends of these nerve branches, and that causes a group of muscle fibers to contract. As a result, the muscle becomes shorter and tenser. When the electrical impulses cease, the fibers stop contracting and the muscle expands and relaxes. Muscle fibers are either completely contracted or completely relaxed; that is not true of muscles. The extent to which a muscle contracts or relaxes depends on the proportion of its muscle fibers that are contracted at a given time. A muscle in which only 25 percent of its fibers are contracted is more relaxed than a muscle in which 75 percent of its fibers are contracted.

Even when your muscles are relaxed, a few muscle fibers remain contracted. These contracted fibers produce a residual tension that, though slight in itself, may be the critical difference between wakefulness and sleep. Dr. Jacobson felt that by repeatedly practicing a relaxation technique, you could virtually eliminate residual muscle tension.

Before you try to use the relaxation method, you should learn to distinguish between tense and relaxed muscles, especially their subtler manifestations. Anybody can tell obviously rigid from flaccid muscles. But detecting the finer gradations of muscle tension and relaxation requires more exquisite self-observation. To acquire this ability, perform this brief exercise, after reading all of the instructions.

1. Once you are comfortably seated, fully extend your arms straight ahead, palms facing upward.

2. Place this book on your right palm.

3. Close your eyes.

4. As you maintain this position for approximately twenty seconds, compare the *mounting* tension in both biceps. Ignore the strain in the rest of your arms; just focus on your biceps. Pay special attention to when you *first* detect a difference in tension between your right and left biceps. Concentrate on how these contrasting tensions feel.

5. After twenty seconds, while your eyes are still shut, suddenly flop your right arm onto your lap. (Don't worry about the book's falling.) Keep your left arm extended.

6. Note how the tension in your right bicep quickly dissipates. During the next twenty seconds compare the decreasing tension in your right bicep to the increasing tension in your left bicep.

7. Abruptly drop your left arm onto your lap and gradually feel its bicep become as relaxed as your right one.

8. Notice the residual muscle tension in both biceps. Make sure you can detect what it feels like.

9. After a two-minute rest, repeat steps 1–8. As you do so, focus on how contracted and relaxed muscles feel. Also try to become as adept as possible at identifying muscle tension. The more sensitive you become at detecting subtler states of tension, the better equipped you'll be to perform progressive relaxation.

What Is Progressive Relaxation and Why Does It Work?

This relaxation technique is called "progressive" for two reasons. First, the more you practice it, the more you progress to deeper states of relaxation. Second, the method involves alternately contracting and relaxing muscle groups in a specific progression (viz, right arm, left arm, face, neck and shoulders, chest and back, stomach, buttocks and hips, right leg, and left leg).

If you're trying to relax your muscles in order to sleep, why bother contracting them at all? To answer this question, Dr. Thomas Borkovec studied whether relaxation preceded by muscle contraction induced sleep faster than relaxation without prior muscle contraction. It did. On the average those insomniacs who used only relaxation fell asleep twelve minutes sooner, whereas those who first contracted and later relaxed their muscles dropped off twenty-three minutes sooner. Thus, contracting and relaxing muscles seems to hasten the onset of sleep more than does merely relaxing them.

Why prior muscle contraction should facilitate sleep is uncertain. Dr. Jacobson felt that by initially contracting muscles you could later achieve a deeper state of relaxation. This highly plausible notion was recently dispelled however. By measuring muscle tension with an electromyograph, doctors have shown that the same level of relaxation can be attained whether or not it is preceded by muscle contraction.

A more likely explanation for why contraction with relaxation hastens the onset of sleep may lie in the *perception* of relaxation. By first contracting your muscles, you can better appreciate subsequent relaxation and residual tension. Being more aware of tension, you can then eliminate it, and thereby *feel* more relaxed.

For the sake of clarity, I have until now written as if muscle tension were initially greater among insomniacs than among noninsomniacs. But contrary to common sense, recent investigations demonstrate that, *as a group*, insomniacs do not exhibit any more tension on their EMGs than do noninsomniacs. Moreover, after relaxation, there is no correlation between the decline of muscle tension and the degree of improved sleep. Relaxation does lower muscle tension. But by itself, reduced tension does not account for the faster onset of sleep that progressive relaxation brings. So if the muscle tension of typical insomniacs is not greater at the outset, and if the success of sleep-induction with relaxation is not related to the extent of diminished muscle tension, then why is progressive relaxation effective at all?

Nobody knows. Dr. Thomas Borkovec has speculated that the self-generated monotony of applying a relaxation method might be the critical sleep-promoting factor. He might be correct. But I'd suggest another, or at least a complementary, explanation: namely, that when focusing on relaxation, your mind is distracted from sleep-preventing thoughts, which then enables you to appreciate more fully the soothing, soporific experience of having relaxed muscles. In short, your *perception* of being exquisitely relaxed is heightened. Regardless of what an EMG reveals, if you feel more relaxed, you are better prepared psychologically to drift asleep.

Even though not all insomniacs are excessively tense, some are. What's more, progressive relaxation helps some people more than others. Consequently, there must be a subgroup of those with chronic nonspecific insomnia who especially benefit from relaxation techniques. Dr. Peter Hauri suggests that this group includes those who have any one (or more) of the following characteristics. (a) They are highly anxious. (b) They have increased muscle tension, or at least feel unusually tense. (c) They take over an hour to fall asleep, but once asleep, they slumber without interruption.* If you show any of these traits, you are most likely to be helped by progressive relaxation. But since Dr. Hauri himself emphasizes that his findings are tentative, it could be that even if you do not meet any of these three criteria, you could still profit from progressive relaxation.

Learning Progressive Relaxation

You will *want* to apply progressive relaxation for the rest of your life. The ability to relax profoundly can not only vanquish insomnia, but also squelch anxiety before stressful events.

Becoming highly proficient at progressive relaxation demands time and persistence. If you are seeking an instant cure for sleeplessness, forget about relaxation. Learning to relax—and I mean *really* relax—requires practice twice a day, every day, for at least a month. Each practice session will last up to twenty minutes. (Later on it will take only five minutes.) Given all the hours you now squander lying awake at night, performing forty minutes of refreshing relaxation exercises a day is well worth the time and effort.

Consistency, not quantity of practice, is most important. Performing ten practice sessions every fourth day is not as useful as conducting two every day.

Before you actually begin to practice this technique, read the rest of this chapter. It is important to have an overview of the method and to be fully acquainted with its details before starting.

To learn progressive relaxation, start by executing its basic unit, the *tension-relaxation sequence*. Begin with your right hand. (If you are left-handed, use your left hand. If

---

*While investigating biofeedback-induced relaxation for imsomniacs, Dr. Hauri found that these criteria predicted a favorable outcome. In the absence of further research, I'm assuming these characteristics also predict who is most likely to fall asleep quickly with other relaxation methods, such as progressive relaxation.

you're ambidextrous, take your pick.) Initiate a tension-relaxation sequence by quickly making an extremely tight fist. Tense these muscles as hard as you can without cramping them. Keep your fist clenched for seven seconds. (To approximate this time, count, "one thousand one, one thousand two, one thousand three, one thousand four, one thousand five, one thousand six, one thousand seven.") Carefully survey each muscle in every finger and make sure that it is as tense as possible.

After rigidly contracting your hand for seven seconds, suddenly release all the tension from your hand. For the next thirty seconds allow all the tension to flow from your muscles so that they relax completely and totally. Imagine the tension leaving your finger tips. Enjoy the relaxation. Relish the tranquility that comes to pervade your entire hand. Midway through this relaxation phase, carefully scrutinize each muscle in every finger to detect any residual tension. If tension lingers in your hand, relax it further. Repeated practice will be necessary to achieve your goal of fully relaxing your muscles.

After thirty seconds of hand relaxation, you've completed a single tension-relaxation sequence. Because the entire progressive relaxation technique is composed of individual tension-relaxation sequences, it is essential to master these sequences. Therefore, repeat this tension-relaxation sequence several times on your right (or left) hand.

Once you understand how to perform this tension-relaxation sequence, you are ready to practice similar sequences for the specific muscle groups involved in progressive relaxation. For the sake of convenience, I have divided the body's skeletal muscles into nine groups. Practice sessions will shortly begin with two tension-relaxation sequences on each of these nine groups in the following order: right arm, left arm, face, neck and shoulders, chest and back, stomach, buttocks and hips, right leg, left leg. Remember, each tension phase will last seven seconds and be succeeded by a thirty-second relaxation phase. Don't worry about the exact timing; approximations will do. In practicing tension-relaxation sequences, pay special attention to the following guidelines.

1. RIGHT ARM (*"Right arm" refers to all the muscles in your right hand, forearm, and upper arm. If you're left-handed, start with your left arm.*)

Tension phase: Place your arm in any comfortable position and then quickly tighten your entire right arm. (Avoid contracting any other muscles in your body.) Your fist should be clenched. Make sure to tense your thumb. Your wrist should be taut. Do not overlook the muscles in your forearm; note what they feel like when contracted. Keep your elbow rigid. Your biceps and triceps—the muscles in the front and back of your upper arm respectively—should be completely tightened. Systematically review each muscles in your right arm to insure that they're as taut as possible. As you increase muscular tension, beware of cramping your muscles or of hurting yourself by straining excessively.

Relaxation phase: Quickly release the tension from all the muscles of your right arm. When you do so, your arm should plop to your lap, chair, bed, or whatever. Make sure every muscle is fully relaxed. Study the relaxation. Feel it. Enjoy it. You may wish to briefly move or shake your arm, or parts of it (especially your fingers), in order to further discharge tension. As you feel the tension flowing from your arm, survey every muscle, starting with your triceps and going straight down to your finger tips, to make sure each one is fully relaxed. The more you relax, the more a pleasant sensation comes over your arm.

2. LEFT ARM (*Now apply the instructions for the right arm to your left arm.*)

3. FACE (*"Face" refers to all the muscles of your scalp, forehead, eyelids, nose, lips, tongue, cheeks, jaw, and chin.*)

Tension phase: Abruptly tense every face muscle. Your eyelids should be shut so tight that you feel the muscles around them being squeezed. Contract your tongue. Wrinkle your nose. Purse your lips. In tensing your jaw, bite down only on your back teeth (to avoid chipping your front teeth).

Beware of straining and therefore hurting your neck. Experience the tension, especially around the curves of your face. Because the face consists of more muscles than any other group, be very careful to make sure that every muscle is fully contracted. Further tighten those that are not already completely tensed. Imagine your face turning into granite, like Mount Rushmore.

Relaxation phase: Exhale when you simultaneously discharge all the tension from your face. Every time you exhale, feel the tension streaming out of every one of your muscles. Think of inhaling as a way of setting the stage for exhaling, which in turn facilitates the further release of tension. Your eyelids should droop so that they lightly, but completely, cover your eyes. Your tongue should rest on the bottom of your mouth. As your jaw relaxes, your mouth will be partly opened. Fully note and relish the pleasures of having your facial muscles relax. Review every one of them to eliminate any remaining tension. Try to achieve a state of relaxation in which it feels as if your face is floating.

4. NECK AND SHOULDERS

Tension phase: Because you cannot breathe or swallow with a fully tensed neck, take a deep breath and swallow *before* contracting your neck. Then suddenly freeze your neck and shoulder muscles. They should be rigid. Feel the big muscles on both sides of your neck contract fully. Your neck may shake; that's okay. Immobilize your throat. To heighten the tension in your shoulders, fling them as far backward as possible. You will feel tension across your chest. When squeezing your neck and shoulders, beware of straining them. Don't overdo it. When reviewing each of your muscles to accentuate the tension in them, don't overlook the two muscles running up the back of your neck.

Relaxation phase: If you are sitting up, when you release the tension, let your arms, shoulders, and head droop all the way forward. If you are lying down, let your head, neck, and shoulders fall comfortably onto the bed. If you want to take a deep breath or to swallow, go right ahead; it may relax you further. As you exhale, imagine tension flowing downward, out of your neck and shoulders. Notice feelings of warmth and heaviness flooding over your upper back, shoulders, neck, and head. Enjoy this growing sense of relaxation.

5. CHEST AND BACK

Tension phase: Before tensing your chest and back, take in a deep breath, hold it a second, and then slowly let it out. After you've exhaled two-thirds of the way, suddenly tense all your chest and back muscles. When you contract your chest muscles, you will be unable to breathe. Don't worry about this; it will only be for seven seconds. Constrict those pectorals. Squeeze in your rib cage. Stiffen your spine. Check each muscle to make certain it is as tight as possible. All four sides of your chest should feel compressed.

Relaxation phase: Abruptly relax your chest and back as you finish exhaling. Then inhale deeply and breathe out gradually. As you exhale this time, note the wave of relaxation flowing through your muscles. Although you cannot actually feel muscle fibers, imagine that every little fiber in your chest and back is expanding. Survey the muscles of your chest and back, spotting and eliminating any lingering tension.

6. STOMACH

Tension phase: As you did when you tightened your chest muscles, take a deep breath and partially exhale before contracting your abdomen. To tense your stomach, squeeze it in so that your entire abdomen feels compressed into a ball.

Relaxation phase: Quickly relax your stomach and complete exhaling. Then take a deep breath, and as you slowly exhale, feel your abdominal muscles relaxing. When they seem to be totally relaxed, relax them some more.

7. BUTTOCKS AND HIPS

Tension phase: Contract every muscle in your buttocks and hips. Don't forget to squeeze the muscles on both the right and left sides and on the bottom of your behind. Make sure you're constricting your buttocks and not your stomach.

Relaxation phase: If you're sitting, it is harder to relax your buttocks and hips fully; do the best you can. If you're lying down, release all the tension. It will take practice to feel these muscles relax completely.

8. RIGHT LEG (*"Right leg" refers to all the muscles in your right thigh, knee, calf, ankle, foot, and toes.*)

Tension phase: Because muscles in the calves and feet are prone to cramping, when you first practice contracting them, gradually increase the tension until they feel taut, yet not uncomfortable. Once you are aware of how tightly your leg muscles will constrict without harm, it will be easier to squeeze your entire leg fully, quickly, yet reassuringly. In contracting your right leg, feel the tension in the front, sides, and back of your thigh. When tightening your calf and foot, bend your ankle and toes upward, so that the latter are pointing to your knee. Make sure to squeeze both the higher and lower parts of your calf. Your knee and ankle should be rigid. As much as possible, tighten your foot and spread your toes. Because so many muscles are involved, systematically review all of them, making certain they are fully tensed. Each leg contains about 20 percent of the total mass of your body's muscles. That's a lot of territory; don't leave any spot uncontracted.

Relaxation phase: Suddenly relax your entire leg and feel the tension leave every muscle. At times, relaxation can be facilitated by briefly wiggling your toes or by shaking other parts of your leg. Let all the tension escape. Eventually your leg will be so relaxed that it will feel like a heavy blob. When your leg seems fully relaxed, carefully survey every muscles to detect and alleviate any residual tension. Study and enjoy the relaxation as it spreads from the top of your thigh to the tips of your toes.

9. LEFT LEG (*Now apply the directions for the right leg to the left leg.*)

Using Progressive Relaxation

Having become acquainted with the components of progressive relaxation, you now are prepared to put the whole technique together.

In planning to use progressive relaxation, arrange for an appropriate time and a suitable place to practice twice a day. Since your attention should be devoted exclusively to the exercises, conduct them under nondistracting conditions. You can't pay full attention to relaxation if your spouse is wandering around the room, the stereo is blasting, or the telephone is ringing. Isolate yourself from these annoyances: Ask your spouse to disappear (for only twenty minutes), shut off the stereo, and take the phone off the hook. Do not sandwich practice sessions between pressing appointments. If you know that immediately after you practice you will have to rush off to pick up the kids, you may concentrate on how quickly you can finish the exercise and not on the exercise itself. Give yourself enough time.

Your two daily practice periods, each lasting about twenty minutes, should be carefully scheduled. Allocate specific times for your sessions and stick to those times. For example, you may conduct one session at 10 A.M. and another at either 4 P.M. or 7 P.M. But at least initially, do *not* practice within an hour of bedtime or when you should be asleep, such as in the middle of the night. Whenever possible, reserve the same times for your sessions every day. If you find yourself thinking, "Well I'll practice on the fly," or "I'll do the exercises when I have a chance," you are starting to become haphazard. The next thing you know you'll be skipping practice. Relaxation sessions should become an integral part of your daily routine.

At first, neither session should be conducted in bed, because beds should be used only for sleeping (Chapter 4). If you apply progressive relaxation in bed before you have fully mastered the technique, you're likely to become frustrated, to give up prematurely, and to aggravate your insomnia. Instead, do your practicing either sitting up in a comfortable chair or sofa or lying down on the floor or on huge, overstuffed pillows.

When you begin to practice, do not immediately plunge into the exercise. Rather, first give yourself a minute to unwind. Get comfortable by turning off the lights, loosening tight-fitting clothes, and uncrossing your limbs. Start each session by slowly taking a few deep breaths and gently closing your eyes. Shutting your eyes will help you focus better on relaxation.

If you're worried about falling asleep during your sessions, you may wish to set an alarm or have someone check on you.

To master the progressive relaxation sleep-induction technique, adopt the following routine:

• **Weeks 1 and 2:** Begin each session by performing tension-relaxation sequences *twice* on each of the nine muscle groups. By the end of the second week you will have become reasonably adept at discerning tension and relaxation states in all nine groups.

• **Week 3:** Follow the same routine, but with two major differences. First, perform a tension-relaxation sequence only *once* on each muscle group. Second, when you have finished with your left-leg exercise, perform *one* tension-relaxation sequence on your *entire body*. For seven seconds, contract all nine muscle groups *simultaneously* and then relax your whole body for about sixty seconds. When you tense your entire body, mentally review every muscle group to be sure it is fully contracted. Similarly, when relaxing your body, systematically inspect every muscle to make certain it is fully relaxed. Use the complete minute to achieve the utmost relaxation. Let yourself go. Imagine being suspended in midair. Enjoy this floating experience; cultivate and relish it.

• **Week 4:** Having mastered relaxation of individual muscle groups, you can now bypass them and simply perform *two* total-body tension-relaxation sequences during each session.

• **Week 5 and afterward:** By now you probably will be highly proficient at progressive relaxation and will be ready to apply it at bedtime. It is important, however, to understand what I mean by "highly proficient," because you should not use this technique to induce sleep until you have attained a state of profound relaxation. You have achieved sufficiently deep relaxation if during practice sessions any one (or more) of the following occurs: You (a) fall asleep, (b) become very drowsy, (c) feel warmth, (d) feel heaviness, (e) experience a floating-in-space sensation, (f) feel extreme lightness, (g) tingle, or (h) have a pins-and-needles sensation.

Once you can produce this profoundly relaxed state, you are ready to apply progressive relaxation for overcoming insomnia at bedtime. To do so, when you wish to fall asleep, employ a single total-body tension-relaxation sequence in bed. Prolong the relaxation phase until you drift off. While relaxing, you will feel peaceful, tranquil, and soothed. Let your body drift naturally to sleep. Don't force it; just let it happen. If you don't immediately fall asleep, don't worry about it. Simply enjoy the relaxation; it's the next-best thing to sleep.

Once you are able to fall asleep with progressive relaxation, discontinue your daily practice sessions. But if after four weeks you have not achieved profound relaxation, keep practicing two total-body tension-relaxation sequences twice a day. When you can successfully induce a state of deep relaxation, apply the method at bedtime. The length of time it takes to produce a profoundly relaxed state varies; some people require two weeks, others need six or more weeks. If you're still not successful by the end of the sixth week, don't despair; just turn to the next chapter.

This entire progressive relaxation routine and schedule is summarized in Table 5.1. As you use this method, you may wish to monitor its effectiveness by continuing to fill out your daily-progress chart (Table 3.2).

Although nearly everyone finds profound relaxation an extremely pleasant experience, a few do not. On rare occasions, patients who are deeply relaxed feel overwhelmingly anxious or depressed; they become restless or scared, or at times, cry or twitch uncontrollably. Why these symptoms occur is unknown. But in these few individuals deep relaxation produces, in all likelihood, an altered state of consciousness in which strong unconscious emotions erupt. If

5.1 / SUMMARY OF PROGRESSIVE RELAXATION TECHNIQUE

WEEK	WHEN	MUSCLE GROUPS*	TOTAL BODY
#1	Daytime or early evening	X 2	0
#2	Daytime or early evening	X 2	0
#3	Daytime or early evening	X 1	X 1
#4	Daytime or early evening	0	X 2
#5+	Bedtime†	0	X 1

TIMING	MUSCLE GROUPS*	TOTAL BODY
Tension	7 seconds	7 seconds
Relaxation	30 seconds	60 seconds, except for the final relaxation phase of a session, which should persist until you end the session or fall asleep

*Order of Muscle Groups:
1. Right arm
2. Left arm
3. Face
4. Neck and shoulders
5. Chest and back
6. Stomach
7. Buttocks and hips
8. Right leg
9. Left leg

†*Signs of Profound Relaxation:* Use progressive relaxation only at bedtime when you have achieved any one (or more) of the following during practice sessions. You:
1. fall asleep
2. become very drowsy
3. feel warmth or heaviness
4. experience a floating-in-space sensation or extreme lightness
5. experience a tingling or pins-and-needles sensation

you repeatedly experience these rare "side effects" of progressive relaxation, I'd suggest you abandon using the technique. That these symptoms emerge at all illustrates how powerful progressive relaxation can be, and that, like sleeping pills, even natural sleep-inducing methods can have adverse consequences.

If, after you have overcome sleeplessness with progressive relaxation, insomnia should reemerge, start the entire routine again. Patients who have successfully employed progressive relaxation for sleep usually say that it works much better the second time around.

Although the precise method outlined in this chapter is an easy and effective way to learn progressive relaxation, you may prefer to use tape-recorded instructions as a way of mastering this technique. I would suggest, however, that you first employ the method described here. But if it would help to hear the instructions recited by a soothing voice, you or a friend can make your own tape recordings by a verbatim reading of the directions in Appendix B.

When anticipating any kind of stressful situation, you may wish to perform a single total-body tension-relaxation sequence. In a minute you will feel calm, relaxed, and confident. Anxiety will not control you; you will control it. But to use "mini-relaxation" at a moment's notice, you must first have mastered the entire progressive relaxation technique.

In the next chapter you will build on this basic method. For now, start practicing, avoid shortcuts, and look forward to a relaxing night's sleep.

CHAPTER SIX

Calming Your Mind

Diana: Going to sleep is like being a garbage disposal. When I go to bed, a lot of garbage stuffs my mind, and until I dispose of it, I can't fall asleep.

Jim: When I'm awake, my mind's asleep. When I attempt to sleep, my mind's awake.

Mitch: My creativity soars at bedtime. I create a thousand ways not to sleep.

For Diana, Jim, and Mitch, sleeping and thinking are incompatible. Plagued by intrusive thoughts, they're unable to sleep. If their insomnia—the triumph of mind over mattress—is to be overcome, they will have to unclutter their minds. But how?

While lying in bed we have all tried to vanquish distracting thoughts by deliberately attempting not to think about them. But this strategy rarely works. Preoccupying thoughts come to resemble unwelcomed house guests: the more you endeavor to get rid of them, the more determined they are to stay. Remember the old gimmick of being told *not* to think about something? For example, I might say, "*Don't* think about Howard Cosell." Until that moment Howard Cosell was probably the last person on your mind. That's no longer so; despite instructions to the contrary, you're now thinking about him. Though "everybody" knows that you can't *force* yourself *not* to think about something, that's precisely what many insomniacs try to do when attempting to sleep.

Unless you're an experienced meditator, you cannot think about nothing. You may, however, replace thoughts of Howard Cosell with something else—let's say your favorite Cole Porter melody or some family tribulation. But now it is Cole Porter or your family troubles rather than Howard Cosell that keeps you awake. It doesn't matter what the thoughts are, as long as they are not conducive to sleep, sleep remains elusive. If you're distracted from sleeping by such intrusive thoughts, you need an approach that at once controls thoughts and induces sleep.

You've already seen how relaxation can help you drift asleep. But whereas progressive relaxation reduces muscle tension *directly,* it affects thinking only *indirectly.* If your insomnia stems primarily from the feeling of increased muscle tension, progressive relaxation by itself should be a sufficient remedy. On the other hand, if bothersome thoughts are the principal barriers to sleep, then methods that *directly* alleviate distracting thoughts may be a necessary supplement to progressive relaxation.

There are several additional circumstances under which progressive relaxation by itself will not induce sleep. In the preceding chapter I emphasized that you should not use relaxation at bedtime until you have achieved a state of profound relaxation. But despite weeks of practice, some people never reach the depth of relaxation that is necessary in order to fall asleep promptly. There also are those who, although they attain profound relaxation during practice sessions, are still unable to sleep by using progressive relaxation. I further indicated that an occasional individual becomes unusually anxious or depressed while in deep relaxation, and that he or she should not try to drift asleep by entering a state of profound relaxation.

Nevertheless, *everyone* can produce, and be comfortable in, a state of *moderate* relaxation. An advantage of the mind-calming techniques explained in this chapter is that they can be used successfully while you are only moderately relaxed. This chapter will present three such mind-calming methods. Deciding which of them will be of most help to you may depend less on *what* you think than on *how* you think.

Verbalizers and Sensers

Ed and Mike gazed at the televised, violent demonstrations outside the 1968 Democratic National Convention in Chicago. Ed wondered aloud if the police had instigated the riots and whether the confrontation would harm Humphrey's chances for the nomination. Ed was outraged and disgusted.

Mike, by contrast, was preoccupied. He could almost feel the clubbings, smell the gas, and taste the blood. To Mike, screams of anguish were heard less from the television set than from inside himself.

Ed is a *verbalizer*, Mike a *senser*. Both were equally horrified. They differed, however, in the *ways* they thought about what horrified them. Even when they look at the same event, Ed's thoughts are primarily rational and Mike's are primarily emotional. Whereas Ed's rely on intellectual analysis, Mike's depend on vivid imagery. As a history professor, Ed reflexively thinks in terms of ideas. As a choreographer, Mike automatically uses his refined sense of sight, sound, and touch to synthesize information. Ed thinks by articulating, Mike by experiencing.

To varying degrees you are primarily either a verbalizer like Ed or a senser like Mike. Which of the two you are has nothing to do with education, intelligence, or mental health. Verbalizing and sensing refers solely to different ways of thinking. By nature you are especially adept at thinking either with linear ideas or with multi-dimensional images. As psychologist Robert Sommer points out, the verbalizer's "intellectual style emphasizes words, concepts, generalities, abstract qualities." He rarely dreams in pictures and almost never in color. The senser thinks by conjuring up rightly detailed sensory creations. His dreams are highly visual and frequently in color. Those with photographic memories are prototypical sensers; mathematicians are prototypical verbalizers.

After first meeting a woman, a verbalizer recounts the experience mainly by describing what was said. A senser recalls mainly the texture of her dress, the inflections of her voice, the color of her eyes, the smell of her perfume, and the grace of her movements. Whereas the senser remembers the conversation by mentally hearing her voice, the verbalizer does so by recounting the content of the exchange.

If you want to determine whether you tend to be a verbalizer or a senser, think of somebody you casually met today for the first time, and note in which way you remember and describe the encounter.

Which of the following sleep-inducing methods are more likely to work for you may depend largely on the *type* of thinker you are. But since everybody thinks both verbally and sensorially, though to different extents, all three of these techniques should be tried. In all probability verbalizers will most effectively use the first method, *soporific phrases,* whereas sensers will best employ *soporific images.* Those of you with both verbalizing and sensing talents will probably get the most mileage out of the third method, *autogenic training.*

Practice will enhance both your verbalizing and sensing capabilities, especially as you apply them to help you sleep. Therefore, don't be discouraged if you don't immediately fall into a deep sleep when you first use these techniques. Time is on your side. As is the case in developing any skill, the longer you work at it, the more proficient you become at it.

Calming Your Mind: Preparatory Steps

Psychologists have proven that the following three techniques calm your mind and induce sleep; but because they are used with progressive relaxation, their effectiveness hinges on the prior mastering of relaxation. You don't have to become the mahatma of relaxation, but you should be reasonably adept at placing yourself into a moderately relaxed state.

All of the following methods should be employed during the relaxation phase of your total-body tension-relaxation sequence. In other words you will apply these mind-calming approaches while still relaxing. They dovetail so nicely that you will soon discover that progressive relaxation and mind-calming techniques are mutually enriching; you may not want to perform one without the other.

All of the preparations and guidelines that you adopted for practicing progressive relaxation apply when you use these mind-calming methods. Continue to set aside two free time slots for practice sessions. If possible, conduct your exercises at the same times every day, so that they become integral parts of your daily routine. Do not apply a technique within an hour of bedtime or when you should be asleep, until you have fully mastered it. Practice in a quiet and tranquil setting. Use a comfortable chair or, if you prefer, the floor—anything but the bed. Make sure your clothes don't feel tight; remove your shoes, if you wish. Be patient; only time and repetition generate results. Finally, in learning these methods, read and, if necessary, reread all of the instructions for a particular technique before you apply them.

Soporific Phrases

What if your mind begins to wander when trying to concentrate on relaxation? Maybe you get bored. Maybe a tune pops into your head. Maybe a chandelier plummets into a spinach salad. Maybe you recall a squabble with your fifteen-year-old. If you *never* become distracted, you're dead. Roving thoughts are inevitable. By employing soporific phrases, however, you can take these distractions in stride, quickly refocus on relaxation, and induce sleep.

Autosuggestion and thought modulation are the "active ingredients" in using soporific phrases. To varying degrees we're all suggestible. Because of the term's pejorative connotations, we don't like to think of ourselves as being suggestible. But suggestibility and gullibility are different. The suggestible person may know who or what is influencing him, the gullible person does not. Being suggestible can be a highly desirable quality, especially if *you* are doing the suggesting. By employing soporific phrases, you capitalize on your own suggestibility in order to foster sleep.

When unwanted thoughts stubbornly lodge in your mind, you need to control them instead of allowing them to control you. Otherwise sleep remains elusive. You will discover, however, that by switching from one soporific phrase to another as soon as you become the least bit distracted, you can keep your attention on sleep-inducing thoughts. By deliberately regulating your thoughts in this manner, you're not going to become annoyed or flustered by every little distraction. You'll be amazed at how long you can, with practice, concentrate on falling asleep. But if autosuggestion and thought modulation are to help you sleep, you need to use the proper soporific phrases in the most effective way.

Like many of us Dorothy Parker tried reciting phrases in order to doze off. She asked, "How do people go to sleep? I'm afraid I've lost the knack. I might try busting myself smartly over the temple with the nightlight. I might repeat to myself, slowly and soothingly, a list of quotations beautiful from minds profound; if I can remember any of the damn things." I suspect she picked the wrong phrases. Helpful soporific phrases should be productive neither of wit nor of wisdom, but of sleep. They should be short, positively worded, simple to remember, and soothing.

There are four types of useful soporific phrases. These are either *muscle* or *mind* phrases consisting of either *statements* or single *words*. Examples of each type are:

1. *Muscle Statements*
   "My body is getting heavier."
   "My left leg is becoming warm."
   "My chest is becoming relaxed."

2. *Muscle Words*
   "Heavy"
   "Warm"
   "Relax"
3. *Mind Statements*
   "I am at peace."
   "I am calm."
   "I am beginning to sleep."
   "I will soon be asleep."
4. *Mind Words*
   "Peace"
   "Calm"
   "Tranquil"
   "Sleep"

There is nothing magical about these particular phrases. My patients happen to prefer them; with practice you'll discover your own favorites. Regardless of the exact phrases you eventually employ, the following routine is a good way to begin. Try it first and improvise later.

Always use soporific phrases during the relaxation phase of a total-body–tension-relaxation sequence. While relaxing moderately, start to recite mentally any of the muscle statements (e.g., "My face is getting heavier."). Continue to repeat, slowly and inwardly, this same phrase. When you *first* become distracted, switch to a mind statement (e.g., "I am at peace."). Continue reiterating this phrase, and when you again become the least bit distracted, quickly refocus your thinking on a muscle word (e.g., "warm"). Keep saying "warm" to yourself until your concentration wanes. At this point switch to a mind word (e.g., "sleep"). When your attention wavers, return to reciting a muscle statement, and so forth, until your mind is calm enough to fall asleep.

To understand the rationale for applying soporific phrases, don't lose sight of the forest for the trees. The exact wording, frequency, and sequence of phrases are important only to the extent that they facilitate autosuggestion and thought modulation. The best phrases are those that you—

not I nor my patients—find most relaxing. Whether you mentally say a particular phrase three or ten times is irrelevant; what is essential, is that the number of times you repeat a phrase is most tranquilizing for *you*. Similarly, the sequence of phrases you ultimately settle on should be one that best calms your mind and helps you doze off. Only practice will show you which phrases to use, how often, and in what order.

The timing and effortlessness of your switches are more critical than the selection of your phrases. The sole purpose of switching phrases when first becoming distracted is to extend your relaxation without being unduly disturbed by wandering thoughts or boredom. If you switch too rapidly, you'll concentrate more on switching than slumbering. As long as using a particular phrase promotes mental and physical relaxation, there is no reason to change it. But when, and only when, an extraneous thought intrudes, you should comfortably and naturally turn to another phrase. Eventually you'll be on "automatic pilot." You'll not have to think, "Now I have to switch." You'll just do it. Your attention will be devoted exclusively to the pleasurable experience of calming your mind with soporific phrases.

In time you'll discover the best sequence of phrases for you. I've suggested going from a muscle statement, to a mind statement, to a muscle word, to a mind word, and then repeating this cycle. At the start, try this sequence. After some trial and error, you should rearrange the order and types of phrases to suit yourself. You may prefer to stick with muscle statements, switching from "My right arm is warm," to "My left arm is warm," and so on through the other seven muscle groups. You may wish to alternate between muscle and mind statements. I like to switch between muscle and mind words. Single words capture the essence of what I want to do—relax my body and unclutter my mind. Dr. Herbert Benson, author of *The Relaxation Response,* concurs. But he has also observed that some religious individuals relax and quell distracting thoughts best by reiterating the same comforting prayer. It may be "The Lord is my shepherd," or "Hear, O Israel: The Lord our God, the Lord is One,'' or any other prayer that brings solace. In any event, you'll have to find out what phrases and sequences are most soothing for you.

Regardless of the phrases you use, say one phrase every time you exhale. When your breathing and thinking are synchronized, muscle relaxation and mind calming will complement and enrich one another. Not only will your mind and body work in unison, but your recitations will automatically proceed at a pace conducive to sleep.

Don't be alarmed if your body starts to tingle; this simply means that you're effectively relaxing by allowing blood to circulate freely through your muscles. If you feel warm, this also is a sign of success. Biofeedback subjects can deliberately raise their body-surface temperatures up to twenty degrees Fahrenheit by merely thinking about phrases such as ''My body is becoming warmer.'' Impressive, our powers of suggestion!

Reciting soporific phrases can make you feel so relaxed and tranquil that, during practice sessions, you may not want to pull yourself out of this blissful state. I can't blame you. Falling asleep is fine at night, but potentially catastrophic in the afternoon. If it helps to put your mind at ease—and that is what soporific phrases are for—then before your practice sessions set an alarm clock or else have someone check on you.

Each of your twice-a-day practice sessions, including a total-body tension-relaxation sequence and soporific phrases, should last about ten minutes. When and only when you can perform soporific phrases on ''automatic pilot'' should you apply them at bedtime. It may require two to three weeks of rehearsal before you attain the proficiency needed in order to induce sleep. Since beds should be used only for sleeping (Chapter 4), if you become annoyed or frustrated when using soporific phrases in bed, stop reiterating them at night and continue practicing them during the day. You'll get the hang of it; just be patient.

Finally, the use of soporific phrases should be an experience to be enjoyed, not a chore to be endured. Saying to yourself, ''Relax,'' is to make a suggestion, not a command. Don't coerce your mind; work in harmony with it. If switching phrases does not keep your mind from becoming distracted, so what? Civilization will survive. The family jewels haven't been stolen. You will not sprout wings or become a tarantula. You'll simply be distracted for a moment. This happens to everybody. If you get lost on a detour, you can always return to the main highway.

Soporific Images

Whereas verbalizers find soporific phrases most effective, sensers doze off on soporific images. Sensers have told me that soporific phrases work for them only if they picture RELAX, WARM, or CALM emblazoned on large signs. I say "told me," because as a verbalizer I find it difficult to think graphically. Wish I could. Sensers have a remarkable ability, especially with practice, to conjure up amazingly accurate, detailed, and realistic scenes to help them fall asleep. Let me show you how.

All the introductory comments about using soporific phrases apply here. Read this entire section before implementing any of the instructions. Mental pictures are generated during the relaxation phase of a total-body tension-relaxation sequence. Set aside ten minutes for two daily practice sessions, ideally at the same times every day. Use soporific images at bedtime only after you have thoroughly mastered the technique, which might require several weeks of practice.

Studies show that it's easier to create images while relaxing and reclining. Consequently—and conveniently— the effects of progressive relaxation and soporific images potentiate each other. Therefore, only a moderate degree of relaxation is necessary in order to create these mental pictures.

Since lying down is more conductive to evoking images than is sitting up, during practice sessions, use a couch, reclining chair, sofa, cascading pillows, or even the floor— anything but your bed. Just make sure you're relatively horizontal and comfortable.

To induce sleep you will alternate between picturing two different images—a candle and a scene of some sort. The candle will serve as your home base, from which you'll travel to various scenes. Between scenes, however, you will always return to visualizing the candle.

Scenes can be anything you want them to be. They can be realistic, such as lying on a beach. They can be fanciful, such as floating on a cloud. Whichever they are—and they can be both—you ought to have created them in detail *before* you employ them. You should not have to fiddle around generating images while practicing. Writing out your scenes in advance will help you detect and fill in missing details; it will also make it easier for you to remember all the particulars of the scenes during practice sessions.

To create hypnotically effective scenes, think of situations, real or illusory, that are especially restful and soothing for you. A scene might involve your stretching out beside a warm, glowing fireplace on a chilly Vermont evening. It might have you lounging comfortably in a hot tub. Or, you might be sprawled on top of a whale that is sprinkling you with water from its snout on a sunny afternoon. While being cooled off, you may choose to have the Champagne Music Makers, the Carpenters, or the Berlin Philharmonic orchestrate your scene. They're your scenes; do with them as you like, and feel free to let your imagination take flight.

Your scenes should be three-dimensional and contain detailed information from, if possible, all five senses—sight, sound, smell, taste, and touch. Richly elaborate images are more engrossing than sparse ones. So embellish your scenes. For example, you might write down and later imagine the following scene:

> I'm snuggled in a sleeping bag. It's dawn. A vermilion sun is bursting on the horizon. A few of its rays dance lightly upon my face. A rainbow of yellows, oranges, and purples ascends onto the pale blue sky. To my left, blades of grass glisten with dew, like a forest of sparkling green candles. To my right, crystal clear water gently cascades downstream. Trout beam a

quivering cold radiance onto the brook's surface. The fresh, misty morning scent is wonderful. Minding its own business, a grasshopper leapfrogs over the grass. Across this verdant field there's no one around for miles and miles. I feel warm, secure, cozy, and alive. A brilliant day awaits me.

Note that in this description I was *experiencing* the scene, not merely watching it. Your scenes should not be observed as if you were peering through a telescope. Instead, you should "enter" your scenes as if you were actually there. Consequently, you will not see your whole body. If your scene is at the seashore, feel the sand, hear the waves, smell the air, see the clouds, experience the tranquility, as if you were "on location." Your whole being should be right there on that seashore; you're not in bed, you're on that beach.

The sole reason for creating a detailed scene is so that you can fully immerse yourself in the situation. If you create a sky-diving scene, think of what you would actually experience while gliding through the air. Remember, however, the purpose of a scene is to lull you to sleep. If a sky-diving scene becomes too exhilarating, it will interfere with sleep. Therefore, to avoid becoming overly stimulated, you can alter a scene by blending fantasy with reality and by concentrating on certain details while excluding others. You may focus on the beauty of the mountains, the sensation of floating, and the melodic strains of a string quartet. Why a string quartet would be heard in the middle of the sky is beside the point. It's your scene, and you can compose it in any way you like. Just make sure you ultimately devise scenes that are sufficiently absorbing, relaxing, and sleep inducing. Although I've recommended that you create first-hand accounts of detailed scenes using as many senses as possible, don't feel obliged to do so. Many people prefer unembellished images—of sunning on a beach, for example—because they're easier to create and remember. The only value of multisensory details is that they may help transport you "into" a scene; but if having to recall numerous details becomes distracting, then the whole purpose of using soporific images is defeated.

Bearing all this in mind, you should now create three to five tranquil scenes. When you've done that, you're ready to practice using soporific images.

When you are in a comfortable state of relaxation, start visualizing a lit candle in your mind's eye. As long as you're able to concentrate on relaxation, the flame will be upright. But when you become distracted, the flame will flutter, as if blown by a passing breeze. While watching this flickering flame, breathe deeply, and when you're again concentrating fully on relaxation, imagine the flame returning to its upright position. Like unwanted thoughts, breezes come and go. Think of the flame as an indicator of your concentration as well as a pleasant and peaceful vision. An upright flame means your body is relaxed and your mind is tranquil. When this occurs, you're ready to switch to your first scene.

Continue to experience this scene for as long as you wish. Really get into it. If you become distracted, switch back to watching the flickering candle. When your attention is focused exclusively on the candle, its flame will be upright. Once settled into this relaxed and tranquil state, you can either return to your first scene or proceed to another image. Your choice depends on which one seems more conducive to sleep. (Initially, however, practice experiencing several scenes to discover the one most soothing to you.) If you were really into a particular scene, try to recapture it. If not, move on to a second scene. Once again, should you become distracted, return to the candle. When calm, switch to a peaceful scene. Keep going back and forth, comfortably and naturally, until your mind is tranquil and you're on the verge of sleep. Remember that switching images is only a *means* to help you ward off diverting thoughts; it is not an end in itself.

Experiencing these restful and relaxing scenes will put you in the best possible state of mind for slipping into a gentle slumber. Desired images rather than unwanted thoughts will fill your consciousness. Normally, insomniacs go to bed unprepared for dealing with the restless night before them. By planning your scenes in advance and by learning how to switch effortlessly between the candle and these scenes, however, you'll retire knowing that you've got a well-worked-out system to help you sleep.

Practice is essential to the effective use of imagery. It takes time to discover which scenes are most likely to facilitate sleep. You must also practice learning how to become so fully absorbed in a scene that you can easily drop off to sleep.

A nice benefit of practicing the use of imagery combined with relaxation is the pleasure that the practice itself affords. So write down those scenes, practice, and enjoy.

Autogenic Training

Once you have practiced soporific phrases and images separately, you should try using them together. During relaxation, for example, you could imagine yourself lounging in a hammock on a balmy Caribbean afternoon while you mentally reiterate, "My body is floating." You would follow all the instructions previously described for both techniques. Behavioral psychologists call this joint application of soporific phrases and images *autogenic training*.

A number of scientific studies of autogenic training underscore its effectiveness. Kahn, Baker, and Weiss reported that a year after learning autogenic training, eleven of thirteen chronic insomniacs continued to sleep successfully. (The two remaining subjects dropped out of the investigation prematurely.) This study suggests that autogenic training eliminates insomnia not only in the short run, but also over the long haul.

Using thirty subjects, Nicassio and Bootzin showed that progressive relaxation alone decreased sleep latency by 44 percent, while autogenic training by itself shortened sleep latency by 58 percent. These results were dramatically superior to those observed with insomniacs who received no treatment. Scientifically speaking, their use of a no-treatment "control group" further supports the belief that autogenic training is indeed effective. Moreover, their data suggest that, as recommended here, the application of progressive relaxation *with* autogenic training offers the insomniac a doubly powerful remedy.

Unlike the previous two experiments, which relied solely on the reports of patients, Traub, Jencks, and Bliss employed polysomnographic recordings to verify objectively the influence of autogenic training. All seven of their chronic insomniacs felt they improved tremendously. The polysomnograph revealed that three of the subjects fell asleep substantially quicker and that two of the three significantly increased their delta sleep. Subjectively, they all slept better; objectively, three actually showed more favorable polysomnographic readings. This study is a remarkable demonstration of how you can improve your sleep *physiologically* by simply evoking soporific phrases and images. To my knowledge, no autogenic training experiment has so far yielded discouraging results. I must emphasize, however, that in my experience none of the techniques presented in this chapter can be applied successfully at bedtime without first practicing them for at least two weeks.

All these studies show that, if conducted properly and diligently, autogenic training has repeatedly overcome insomnia in even the most problematical sleepers. Although many word-of-mouth suggestions for vanquishing insomnia may work occasionally, few methods can withstand rigorous scientific scrutiny. Granted, more research is needed, especially polysomnographic studies confirming the value of these mind-calming techniques. Meanwhile, the available evidence provides genuine hope for desperate insomniacs who fear that absolutely nothing will help them sleep.

Speaking of evidence, you may wish to gather some of your own. By continuing to fill out your daily-progress chart (Table 3.2), you can determine if soporific phrases, soporific images, or autogenic training work best for you. Give at least two weeks to each of these methods before you decide how effective they are for you.

Once you have mastered these techniques, you may want

to use them to settle your nerves in *any* anxiety-provoking situation. For example, if you become extremely tense when speaking in front of a group, you may wish to spend a minute or two beforehand mentally reciting the word "peaceful" while simultaneously relaxing your muscles. What's more, the mind-calming program outlined in this chapter has been shown to reduce the stress leading to hypertension, heart attacks, and strokes.

These methods can thus improve your health, calm your mind, and help you drift asleep. But what do you do if you drop off and wake up a few hours later? I'd suggest turning the page to find out.

CHAPTER SEVEN

Overcoming Nighttime Awakenings

Waking up in the middle of the night is a damn nuisance!

Actually, that's not quite true. The problem is not waking up, but staying awake. Almost everybody awakes at least once; many do so five or more times a night. Most people, however, are unaware of ever awakening, because they immediately fall back to sleep. Even middle-of-the-night awakenings lasting up to three or four minutes are often forgotten by morning.

Waking up in the middle of the night and being unable to return to sleep soon is technically known as *middle insomnia*. This problem can be excruciating; it's hellish enough to lie awake, as David Copperfield lamented, "always tossing about like a distressed ship in a sea of bedclothes." But what is particularly exasperating is being utterly helpless to rectify the situation. Having abandoned all hope of getting back to sleep, you feel like a condemned prisoner waiting for dawn.

What's really screwy is that a great deal of the anguish caused by middle insomnia can be disposed of in an instant. Middle insomnia is often as much a problem of outlook as it is of sleep. If you spent all these wakeful nighttime hours

115

entertaining yourself by perusing a novel or by listening to records, your suffering could be virtually eliminated.

The fact is that when you become tired, you'll drop off, and that your body will eventually obtain all the sleep it requires. Except for a few conditions noted below, middle insomnia should not engender despair. If you're plagued by nocturnal awakenings, however, I know from experience that you'll probably feel I'm being dreadfully glib and that you'll not accept this solution.

Barbara was a sixty-seven-year-old practicing attorney who was tormented for eight weeks by middle insomnia. Otherwise, she was in superb health; she displayed a keen intellect and led an active life. Nevertheless, sleeplessness caused her to insist that her universe was collapsing. Barbara readily dozed off at 11 P.M., but an hour later she was awake and frantic. "How can I read or relax when it's the middle of the night? There *must* be something wrong with me. People simply don't lose all this sleep without becoming sick." Although not fatigued during the day, Barbara dismissed my reassurances. "I know you've said that I'm getting enough sleep. But you don't understand—the boredom of lying awake is driving me to distraction."

Actually, I did understand. I knew her distress was genuine; for years I've heard similar tales of futility. I've come to anticipate that comforting words will only fall on deaf ears. The fact remains, however, that Barbara's despondency was not caused by inadequate sleep, but by excessive boredom. She was unable to enjoy her extra waking hours.

If you repeatedly wake up in the middle of the night but do *not* experience fatigue the next day, I hope you will stop worrying about it and start using these extra hours to good advantage. But if your middle insomnia continues to be upsetting, especially if you're tired the following day, your discomfort can still be alleviated. To overcome middle insomnia, you must first understand what may be causing, or at least contributing, to your problem.

Causes of Middle Insomnia

Advancing age and middle insomnia go hand in hand. Although there are wide individual variations, sleep normally lightens with maturity. Starting in the late forties, delta sleep decreases, while stage 1 and nocturnal awakenings increase. Whereas young adults awake, on the average, only once in the middle of the night, sixty-year-olds typically awake five or six times. Although many of the elderly report more than ten awakenings, 20 percent of them sleep straight through the night. Inexplicably, one survey revealed that older women reported twice as many nocturnal awakenings as did elderly men. In summary, those under fifty are more likely to have difficulties falling asleep; those over fifty are more likely to have middle insomnia. Waking up at night, however, is not an inevitable consequence of growing older.

Major depressions are the second-leading cause of continued middle insomnia. People with these types of depressions may feel profoundly down in the dumps *or* be unable to experience pleasure; nothing interests them. Although they may have troubles falling asleep, most often they complain of middle insomnia or of awakening early in the morning and being unable to return to sleep. They frequently suffer from loss of appetite, unintentional loss of weight, difficulties in concentrating, slowed or agitated movements, unreasonable guilt, low self-esteem, or persistent suicidal thoughts. If you have any of these symptoms in addition to insomnia, you must first read the sections on depression in Chapter 10.

You may or may not be suffering from depression. But if you are, rest assured that excellent treatments for depression and the sleeplessness that accompanies it are readily available. If you do have depression, the recommendations for overcoming middle insomnia presented in this chapter will *not* be helpful.

The use of sleeping pills ranks third among the major causes of middle insomnia. By producing REM rebound or by causing a disproportionate amount of light sleep, hypnotics can seriously disrupt sleep in the middle of the night. If you're currently taking any sleeping pills, it's vital for you to read Chapter 9 before you employ any of the methods advanced in this chapter.

Similarly, the following remedies will *not* alleviate middle insomnia caused by sleep apnea, narcolepsy, nicotine withdrawal, nightmares, night terrors, alcohol, or frequent nocturnal urination and pain.

If you frequently awake gasping for air and also snore excessively, you might have an uncommon but serious condition known as *sleep apnea*. If you have these symptoms, you must read about this disorder in Chapter 10 before using any of the suggestions listed below.

Many patients with narcolepsy suddenly have their muscles give out when experiencing a strong emotion. They may abruptly and repeatedly fall asleep during the day for no apparent reason. Less often they hallucinate on drifting asleep or are unable to move on awakening in the morning. Though narcoleptics usually sleep excessively, some of them frequently awake in the middle of the night. If you have any of these symptoms along with middle insomnia, it's imperative that you first read about narcolepsy in Chapter 10. There is good treatment for it, but that treatment does not include the suggestions outlined in this chapter.

Heavy smokers, who arise in the middle of the night craving another puff, should first check out the discussion on nicotine in Chapter 4.

Nightmares and a similar problem called *night terrors* are considered in Chapter 10.

Alcohol use is also notorious for disrupting sleep in the middle of the night. To understand why this happens and what can be done about it, read Chapter 9 and the brief section (pp. 70–71) on alcohol in Chapter 4.

When a specific cause for insomnia can be identified, the only way to overcome that insomnia, is to treat its cause and not merely its symptoms. On the other hand, if you do *not* suffer from depression, hypnotic abuse, sleep apnea, narcolepsy, nicotine withdrawal, nightmares, night terrors, alcohol abuse, or nocturnal physical symptoms—and are nevertheless bothered by nighttime awakenings—this chapter is for you. You'll learn a comprehensive program for successfully preventing and coping with middle insomnia. And it makes sense to start right at the time and scene of the crime—your bed in the middle of the night.

The Big Mistake

It's 2:30 in the morning, and you wake up. Perhaps it's due to a noisy neighbor or possibly to nothing that's obvious. What you do know, however, is that you're awake, and, to put it euphemistically, you're annoyed.

Now you may inadvertently aggravate the situation. You may stare indignantly at the clock, its luminescent face seeming to rub in that it's another four hours till sunrise. You begin to fret. In vain you bury your head beneath a pillow.

Alternatively, you may say, "Oh well," stumble out of bed, and weave your way into the kitchen to gobble down a peanut-butter-and-jelly sandwich. On the way you trip over your slippers, bump into a wall or two, and are momentarily blinded when you turn on the lights. After consuming your sandwich, you're too awake to sleep, and too asleep to be fully awake.

The "big mistake" was that as soon as you realized you were awake, you understandably, but ill-advisedly, increased your arousal. By working yourself into a tizzy, leaving the bedroom, turning on the lights, and eating a sandwich, you unintentionally went from a state of semialertness to total wakefulness. Once again, middle insomnia is not a problem of awakening; this happens nearly every night to almost everyone. The real problem is being unable to fall back to sleep. Alertness and sleep are incompatible. On awakening, the more excited, annoyed, or active you become, the more difficult it is to quickly drop off again. Conversely, the calmer and more relaxed you are after waking up, the easier it is to drift back to sleep.

The exact moment you are first aware of being awake is critical. At this juncture, if you rouse yourself further, this fleeting opportunity for sleep will escape. On the other hand, if you try to maintain your oblivious state, your chances for recapturing sleep are greatly enhanced.

What to Do on Awakening?

The key to knowing how to respond during the critical moment of waking up is self-observation. When you awake repeatedly in the middle of the night, a predictable pattern of thought and behavior emerges. To overcome middle insomnia, you must first identify this pattern.

One of three patterns is likely to develop. First, your muscles may be tense. Having practiced the tension phase of progressive relaxation, you should be adept at quickly discerning this state. Second, your mind may be excessively stimulated—thoughts will be racing or emotions will be escalating. Third, both your muscles and mind may be overactive.

The only way to discover which of these three patterns is yours is to see what happens immediately after you awake. To sharpen the accuracy of your assessment, make these self-observations after several consecutive awakenings, whether they occur on a single evening or over a couple of nights. What transpires during one awakening may be mere happenstance. What you note repeatedly is more likely to be your habitual pattern—and that's what you want to determine. The only pitfall is remembering to make these observations when you first awake. Some people claim it's helpful to write a memo to oneself just before retiring. To help her remember, one patient of mine puts a snug rubber band on her wrist just before going to bed.

Once you've identified the pattern, you're ready to carry out a solution. (Put off starting, however, until you've read this entire chapter.) The very first thing to do on waking up is to stay put, stay calm, and stay relaxed. Don't make that "big mistake" of unnecessarily increasing your arousal. Slowly say to yourself, "I'm, calm, relaxed, and sleepy."

Your arousal-response pattern determines your next step.

If your muscles are tense, relax them thoroughly. You should *not* tense your muscles as you did with progressive relaxation; that will stimulate arousal. Just place yourself into a deep state of total-body relaxation. Review all nine muscle groups to expel any residual tension. Remain calm, and let your relaxed body float you back to sleep.

If your mind is overactive, immediately employ soporific phrases, images, or autogenic training—depending on which technique has previously worked best for you. When applying any of these methods after a nocturnal awakening, exert as little thought, concentration, and effort as possible. Stick to one phrase or to one image. Don't complicate matters by shifting phrases or images whenever you become distracted. If you become momentarily diverted, just take it in stride. By simplifying things you'll minimize arousal. Particularly suitable phrases for overcoming middle insomnia are "I will remain calm," "I will soon be asleep," "I am still relaxed," and "sleepy." The flickering candle is an ideal image.

If, after awakening, your mind is stirred *and* your muscles are tight, apply both soporific phrases (or images) *and* relaxation.

The purposes of using relaxation and soporific-phrase and -image techniques vary with the time when they are used. As discussed in the previous two chapters, when these methods are employed to help you initially fall asleep, their goal is to create a soothing climate for sleep. When carried out following nocturnal awakenings, their purpose is to prevent further arousal. It's easier to fall asleep when you're half-awake as opposed to fully awake. Hence, for overcoming middle insomnia, these techniques are intended to contain and retain this half-awake state so that your arousal does not escalate to the point where sleep becomes irretrievable.

On awakening, you will be a little groggy. That's good— you want to be groggy. The groggier you are, the easier it will be to return to sleep. Using relaxation and soporific-phrase and -image methods must not clear up that grogginess. If they do, stop! Just let yourself doze off naturally.

Using these techniques in the middle of the night to

minimize arousal requires practice. It's unlikely that you will be able to successfully implement these approaches during the first several nights you try them. It takes time to learn how to apply these methods calmly and swiftly as soon as you wake up.

You cannot develop these skills in the afternoon; you can do so only when you awake at night. But it does help to plan in advance what methods you're going to employ if you do awake prematurely. Once you have determined if you habitual pattern on waking up is to have tense muscles, an overactive mind, or both, there's no reason to be self-observant every time you wake up. After you've chosen a technique, when you awake in the middle of the night, you should not have to worry about when to switch phrases, what images to experience, or how tense your leg is. Your immediate goal is to prevent further arousal. Applying these techniques is simply a means to this goal, not the goal itself. If you can limit arousal and stay groggy, you'll be asleep in no time flat.

What to Do If You're Still Awake?

Let's say that, despite your best efforts, alertness overcomes grogginess. You've tried relaxing your body and calming your mind to contain arousal—all to no avail.

If fifteen minutes or so have elapsed and you're still awake, then it's time to use relaxation with or without soporific phrases and images—just as you learned to do in Chapters 5 and 6. The only departure is that, once again, you do not tense your muscles, but just cultivate relaxation.

Because at this juncture you're reasonably tranquil to begin with, relaxation and mind-calming methods are likely to be effective. Although your attempts at preventing arousal have not been totally successful, neither have their totally failed. If you've kept your cool, haven't panicked, and at least minimized your arousal, you still have a good chance to fall asleep promptly. Be patient and don't get alarmed.

Remember that insomniacs tend to overestimate the duration of their awakefulness in the middle of the night. You may actually be asleep sooner than you think.

Coping with Sleepless Nights

If you're still awake after thirty minutes, it's time to shift gears, or rather locations. The critical period of limited arousal has expired. Muscle relaxing and mind calming have come to naught. Worse yet, you're wide awake. Where do you go from here? Into another room, that's where.

In Chapter 4 I explained that if you become accustomed to lying in bed, frantic and unable to sleep, you psychologically link being in bed with being frustrated. Consequently, if you are to sleep in bed, you may have to sever that negative emotional link. To do so, I suggested that if you can't *initially* doze off in fifteen minutes, you should leave the bedroom. Only when you are sleepy, should you return to bed.

Although this *stimulus control* technique was devised for solving problems of getting to sleep, it can be equally useful for coping with middle insomnia. The psychological principle on which the technique rests is applicable to both situations. You can learn to detest the bed as much in the middle of the night as at its outset.

If you've tried relaxing and mind-calming techniques for thirty minutes without success, you should go into another room. Engage in a low-keyed, pleasant activity, such as watching an old movie on television or reading a new *National Geographic* feature. Only when you are on the verge of sleep should you return to bed. If you fall asleep, great! But if you're still awake after fifteen minutes, leave the bedroom again. Keep following these guidelines until you finally drift off.

Although sticking religiously to this stimulus control protocol yields excellent results, you may be reluctant to climb out of bed, hoping that eventually you'll be knocked out by sheer exhaustion. Remaining in bed, however, will only increase your frustration, feed your hostility toward the bed, and sap your energy.

You might want to stay in bed, feeling there's always a chance, however remote, that you'll get some shut-eye. Anything, I guess, is possible. But after weeks of tossing and turning, what are the chances that on *this* night you'll fall asleep by remaining in bed? Zilch! Staying in bed is wishful thinking; stop wishing and start thinking. When you're sufficiently tired, you'll fall asleep.

Even if you believe that using this stimulus control method is sound advice, boredom may prevent you from taking it. Often it is difficult to find and perform activities while waiting for sleep. I wish there were a simple formula for coping with boredom. There isn't. One person's excitement is another's monotony. The only one who really knows what interests you is *you*.

The following principles for dealing with being awake at night may nevertheless be useful.

• *If you're bored, admit it*. Near the beginning of this chapter, I recounted Barbara's discomfort with middle insomnia and *insomnophobia*. The latter term, which I coined during a sleepless night, refers to an irrational fear of not getting sufficient sleep. Intellectually, Barbara knew that eventually she would obtain enough sleep. But emotionally, waking up repeatedly in the middle of the night convinced her that she "must be sick." Having nothing to do, she remained up and stewed over her mysterious "illness." It was difficult for Barbara to accept that her inability to entertain herself at night was primarily responsible for keeping her awake. Once she came to recognize this, however, she was able to attack her boredom directly and constructively. Therefore, if you're bored at night, face it so you can deal with it.

• *Plan your nighttime activities in advance*. If you awake in the middle of the night, you're apt to be frustrated, exhausted, and irritable. Your lack of energy will be due not only to being awake at an unseemly hour, but also, as you'll see in the next chapter, to the possibility that you're at a low point in your circadian cycle. Feeling so discombobulated, you may have trouble simply deciding how to amuse yourself until you fall asleep. Now you're experiencing a double disappointment—you can't sleep and you can't find anything satisfying to do. But if you plan nighttime activities during the day, when you're fully alert and more at ease, you'll be better prepared to contend with middle insomnia. It's comforting to know that you have an agenda to turn to in case you awake prematurely. Possessing this reassurance may, in and of itself, help you sleep.

• *Be creative in planning a nighttime agenda*. View boredom not as an inevitable punishment, but as a creative challenge. While preparing your nighttime activities, let your imagination blossom. Make a list of all those things you have always wanted to do but for some reason have never done. Brain storm with friends.

Don't immediately rule out suggestions simply because they can't be performed at night; implausible ideas may lead to practical plans. For example, although Barbara had always yearned for a garden, she was not about to plan tomatoes at three o'clock in the morning. But by sticking with the wish for a garden, it dawned on her that she could use her early morning vigils to hatch a horticultural plot. When she was unable to fall back to sleep, she learned about mixing fertilizers, pruning plants, buying seeds, and the like. She thus stopped worrying about losing sleep, felt proud of this accomplishment, and became so enthusiastic about having a vegetable patch that five months later she reaped her first harvest. In short, by thinking creatively you can develop plans for overcoming nighttime boredom.

Perhaps one of the best examples of planning we owe to Count von Keyserling. He went as far as to commission a "smooth and lively" melody to relieve the tedium of his sleepless nights. As the Russian ambassador to the Dresden court, he turned to his longtime friend and protégé, Johann Gottlieb Goldberg. Being the count's harpsichordist as well as Johann Sebastian Bach's pupil, Goldberg prevailed on his mentor to write the music. Published in 1742, Bach's composition became known as the *Goldberg Variations*, because Goldberg played them to the insomnia-ridden count.

Middle-of-the-night activities are a means and not an end. Their purpose is to make it easier for you to pass the early morning hours until you're sleepy enough to return to bed. Once again, the biggest obstacles to using this stimulus control method are insomnophobia, lack of determination, and boredom. But on recognizing that you *will* obtain sufficient sleep and that you *can* eliminate nighttime monotony, you'll be able to use this technique and reestablish a proper sleep-wake cycle. Depending on how long you've been plagued by middle insomnia, it may take you one or two days, weeks, or possibly months before this stimulus control method has you routinely sleeping through the night. So stick with it and you'll sleep without interruption.

Relaxation, mind-calming, and stimulus control techniques are all used to overcome middle insomnia when you awake at night. But as I've pointed out before, daytime activities also affect sleep significantly. When you apply the following three suggestions in conjunction with those already outlined in this chapter, you'll have a comprehensive and effective program for vanquishing middle insomnia.

Exercise

Consistent daytime exercise increases delta (deep) sleep. Consequently, a regular program of physical fitness is an ideal remedy for middle insomnia.

For best results, exercise in the afternoon or early evening. Morning exercise is performed too early in the day to be an effective soporific. On the other hand, exercising within three hours of bedtime will stimulate your system, thereby making it harder to fall asleep. Therefore, to eliminate middle insomnia, exercise in the afternoon or early evening. For more details, review the section on exercise in Chapter 4.

Reduce Noise

Whether blatantly or subtly, noise disrupts sleep. You are obviously aware of being startled in the middle of the night by thunderstorms, sonic booms, or bellowing traffic. It is less well known that softer sounds lighten the depth of sleep. In the earlier half of the evening, when delta sleep reigns, excessive noise replaces stage 4 with stages 2 and 1 sleep. Consequently, although you remain asleep, you may feel less refreshed the following day. In the latter part of the night, when stage 2 and REM sleep predominate, sounds of moderate intensity may awaken you. But because most people plummet back into sleep almost as soon as they awake, these nocturnal awakenings often go undetected. Even if unnoticed, these "mini-awakenings" hardly restore your body's energy. Therefore, to have an optimal night's sleep, reduce excessive noise.

Amy Lowell, the American poet and critic, was determined that noise would not interfere with her sleep. When lodging in a hotel, she would reserve five rooms—the one she actually slept in and the four above and beside her.

If you want to diminish noise but lack Lowell's flair for the impractical, you might want to review the suggestions outlined in Chapter 4.

Increase Prior Wakefulness

The longer you're awake before retiring, the faster you'll fall asleep and, for present purposes, the deeper you'll sleep. Therefore, anything you can do to expand your prior wakefulness will help you to overcome middle insomnia.

Daytime naps, for instance, should stop, because they sharply reduce prior wakefulness. Moreover, although going to bed early may be a tempting way to catch a few extra winks it has, paradoxically, just the opposite effect. Since retiring prematurely decreases prior wakefulness, you'll have more problems both drifting off and waking up in the middle of the night. Consequently, go to sleep only when you're really tired.

Another means of eliminating middle insomnia by expanding prior wakefulness is to arise earlier in the morning. Nobody likes waking up any sooner than absolutely necessary; then again, nobody relishes nightly awakening. Therefore, if you're continually bothered by middle insomnia, adopt the following routine:

1. Awake an hour earlier than normal. When your alarm rings, make sure that you promptly get up and stay out of bed.

2. If after a week you're still not sleeping through the night despite arising sixty minutes earlier, raise the ante by thirty minutes—that is, if your sleep has not improved markedly by the second week, awake ninety minutes sooner than usual.

3. Keep getting up half an hour earlier for each additional week you're plagued by middle insomnia.

4. When the frequency and length of your nocturnal awakenings are reduced to an acceptable point, begin recouping your sleep by setting your alarm for fifteen minutes later each week.

5. Keep arising an additional fifteen minutes later every week until you return to your normal wake-up time.

6. If middle insomnia again bothers you, awake thirty minutes sooner each week until the problem is under control.

It's odd that less sleep should improve sleep. But a major purpose of sleep is to refresh; to this end, the quality of sleep is as vital as its quantity. A pattern of deeper and more consolidated sleep will restore your energy more quickly and effectively than will a pattern of dragged-out, fragmented sleep. So don't be leery of increasing your prior wakefulness by eliminating naps, going to bed later, and arising earlier.

All through the Night

You don't have to live with middle insomnia; nocturnal awakenings are not ordained by heaven. Whether you've

Comprehensive Program for Overcoming Nighttime Awakenings

1. *Rule out the possibility of*
   A. depression (Chapter 10),
   B. sleep-pill use (Chapter 9),
   C. sleep apnea (Chapter 10),
   D. narcolepsy (Chapter 10),
   E. heavy cigarette smoking (Chapter 4),
   F. nightmares or night terrors (Chapter 10),
   G. alcohol use (Chapters 4 and 9),
   H. physical illness (Chapter 10 and see your doctor).
2. *As soon as you awake in the middle of the night,*
   a. avoid the "Big Mistake"; minimize arounsal, stay put; say to yourself, "I'm calm, relaxed, and sleepy."
   b. if your muscles are tense, employ total-body relaxation without a tension phase (Chapter 5).
   c. if your mind's stirred up, use a single soporific phrase or a simple soporific image (Chapter 6). Don't switch from one phrase (or image) to another. Keep things simple.
   d. if both your muscles and your mind are tense, combine 2b and 2c.
3. *If you're still awake after 15 minutes, apply relaxation and autogenic training techniques as if initially falling asleep (Chapters 5 and 6).*
4. *If you're still awake after 30 minutes,*
   a. leave the bedroom,
   b. perform prearranged nighttime activities, and
   c. return to bed only when sleepy.
5. *Conduct afternoon or early evening physical-exercise sessions (Chapter 4).*
6. *Reduce excessive noise (Chapter 4).*
7. *Increase prior wakefulness by*
   a. eliminating naps,
   b. going to bed only when tired, and
   c. waking up earlier in the morning.
8. *If you're still bothered by middle insomnia,*
   a. read Chapter 8 to see if you have an abnormal circadian rhythm; if you don't,
   b. consult a sleep disorders clinic (Appendix A).

been prematurely waking up for one month or for twenty years, there's no excuse for putting up with this any longer.

Adopting hit-or-miss efforts will not eliminate middle insomnia. Worse yet, by tackling the problem half-heartedly, you risk aggravating your sleeplessness by becoming more and more discouraged and frustrated.

On the other hand, by employing a comprehensive strategy for overcoming middle insomnia, you assure yourself peaceful, uninterrupted sleep. Collectively, the suggestions advanced in this chapter constitute such a program, since they influence all twenty-four hours of your sleep-wake cycle. This plan, which is summarized below, really works. But the only way to obtain the maximum benefit from it is to apply it thoroughly and persistently. To help you do so, you may wish to continue filling out your daily-progress chart (Table 3.2).

If after two months of diligently using this program, you still have middle insomnia, don't give up! Instead, call your nearest sleep disorders clinic (appendix A); by monitoring your sleep with polysomnographic recordings, the staff will be able to uncover your nighttime nemesis.

Before consulting a clinic, however, you should consider the possibility that your middle insomnia is due to an abnormal circadian rhythm. On the other hand, once you have finally succeeded at sleeping through the night, you may be faced with a new problem—getting up. You may be less than ecstatic about relinquishing your valiantly won sleep. But all good things, including blissful slumber, come to an end. Therefore, we now address the two different but often related problems of getting up and of abnormal circadian rhythms.

CHAPTER EIGHT

Getting Up

Oversleeping can be a catastrophe. Always being late for work may put you out of work altogether. When you don't awake on time, you can miss your plane, ruin your vacation, and, if you oversleep consistently, even destroy your reputation.

After trying for three years, Robert finally landed a teaching position at a small private school in New England. But when his students assembled for his very first nine o'clock class, everybody was there, except Robert. He had overslept. Over the next two weeks he was late for most of his classes. The students began to ridicule his tardiness; they even established a betting pool on whether Robert would arrive on time. The principal was not amused. Robert apologized. "I'm terribly sorry, but I'm a 'night person.' I just can't wake up. I've tried everything—even going to bed at eight o'clock so that I could get up on time. But when I did, it took me forever to fall asleep, and I still couldn't wake up on time." Convinced that he was doomed to oversleep, yet realizing his job was on the line, he asked to teach only afternoon classes. The principal denied his request, but gave him one more chance, Robert flubbed it, and was fired.

Did Robert deserve to be dismissed? Probably. But if you have as much difficulty waking up as Robert, you can sympathize with his predicament. Getting up can be an annoying if not agonizing experience. As Pablo Picasso explained, "I understand why they execute condemned men at dawn. I just have to see the dawn in order to have my head roll all by itself."

Picasso was hardly the only person to share Robert's dilemma. In a survey of 600 Florida residents, Dr. Wilse Webb found that 17 percent of them took over an hour before they felt alert. Fewer than 200 felt refreshed on arising, and five out of six people failed to wake up spontaneously. Difficulty in getting up is a widespread problem.

Despite its pervasiveness—and the incalculable loss of work hours, embarrassment, and discomfort resulting from it—the distress that accompanies waking up receives little attention. For example, none of the most widely used medical-student textbooks that discuss sleep address the common problem of getting up in the morning.

On waking up people are, to varying extents, "leapers" or "draggers." Leapers assume that since they can bounce out of bed, everybody else should be able to do the same.

Leapers are puzzled, if not amused, watching draggers compensate for their problem. As you might have guessed, Robert's wife, Mary Rae, was a leaper. When they were first married, she was aghast every morning to find no fewer than five alarm clocks hidden in their bedroom. What amazed Mary Rae even further, was that despite all these clocks, Robert usually would fall right back to sleep. Leapers don't understand draggers; they view them as being either lazy or crazy. Worse yet, draggers often agree; they tend to be envious of leapers and ashamed of themselves.

This chapter is dedicated to the draggers among you. Although the leapers of this world—a privileged minority—are unsympathetic to your plight, you need to know that your predicament is widely shared and very real. Your problem is usually due to biology, not to laziness nor craziness. So don't be ashamed of being a dragger.

If you're a dragger, you *may* become a leaper by using

the information in this chapter. Notice, I said "may" not "will"; effecting this transformation depends on the cause of your difficulties in waking up. What you *can* expect, however, is to understand oversleeping and to awaken with greater ease and vitality. Because biorhythms significantly affect getting up, other sleep and waking problems related to them, such as work shift changes and jet lag, will be addressed in this chapter.

How You Wake Up

Before you say "dreadfully," let's ask what is meant by waking up? Does waking up simply mean opening your eyes? Does it refer to having an awake (stage o) EEG pattern? Or does getting up also include becoming fully alert and functional? In this chapter waking up involves all of these activities.

When you get up is largely influenced by your circadian rhythms, a topic explored later in this chapter. *How* you get up is significantly determined by the sleep stage from which you arise.

If speed of awakening is measured by how soon you open your eyes and show an alert EEG, then you awake more quickly from REM than from any other sleep stage. Otherwise, the deeper the sleep stage from which you're aroused, the longer it takes you to get up. These patterns are not accidental; REM occurs predominately during the early morning hours, while stage 4 takes place primarily during the first half of the night.

You would expect that the sooner you open your eyes and attain an awake EEG, the faster you would be able to perform well on tests of mental agility. But just the opposite is true. Those who arise from stage 4 do best on these tests, whereas those who awake from REM do worst. When studied in a sleep laboratory, subjects awakened from REM squelched an alarm-clock buzzer within a split second, but typically required thirty seconds to clear away their mental cobwebs.

From whatever sleep stage they emerged, their minds were mobilized before their bodies. To test how quickly muscle power recovers after getting up, Dr. Wilse Webb's staff compared the handgrip strength of healthy male college students during the day and on arising. As soon as they awoke, their average strength was 13 percent below par. Two minutes elapsed before their muscle strength returned to normal. Dr. Webb's team also showed that the speed of mental and physical restoration was not influenced by the duration of prior sleep. Whether subjects slept one, five, or eight hours before arising, the results were identical as long as they awoke from the same sleep stage.

If you are slumbering in stage 1, or, to a lesser degree, in stage 2, although technically asleep, you possess some awareness of the outside world. Alpha waves (indicating wakefulness) can momentarily sneak into stage 1 and, less often, into stage 2 EEG patterns. Consequently, you not only can awake more readily from these stages, but you're more apt to do so when cued by subtle external stimuli. I often sit across from a man in the subway who appears sound asleep. But when the train pulls up to the 59th Street stop, he suddenly awakes, like an automaton, snatches his briefcase, and vanished into the station. He's probably arising from light sleep.

Although it's been known since antiquity that you're likely to awake from a dream, the explanation for this has changed, at least superficially. Around 200 A.D. the Latin Church Father Tertullian observed, "They say that dreams are more sure and clear when they happen towards the end of the night, because then the vigor of the soul emerges, and heavy sleep departs." In our more secular society, this common phenomenon of waking up from a dream is ascribed to the predominance of REM during the latter portion of sleep. These religious and scientific explanations, however, are not as divergent as they might appear. If REM dreaming is the modern equivalent of the "vigor of the soul," then Tertullian was remarkably insightful.

Arising from REM sleep can be a mixed blessing. Although you quickly open your eyes, you may not want to.

After all, the possibility of holding onto a fascinating dream is more alluring than the prospect of brushing your teeth. On the other hand, if an exciting day awaits you, greeting it will in all likelihood take precedence over retaining an engrossing dream. The ease and speed of a REM awakening are influenced by what you get up to as well as by what you get up from.

At times, awakening from REM sleep may be amusing, troubling, or frightening. Even if they're not arising from an erotic dream, men of all ages are likely to have an erection. Erections normally accompany REM sleep.

If you wake up seeing unreal images or hearing illusory sounds or voices, don't be alarmed. These experiences, known as *hypnopompic hallucinations*, are merely remnants of REM sleep that persist into wakefulness. Just as alpha rhythm can intrude into stage 1 and 2 sleep, so REM patterns can slip into stage o (waking). Arising to hallucinations does *not* mean you're psychotic. It does mean you're biologically endowed with the capacity to dream momentarily soon after awakening. Hypnopompic hallucinations are nothing to worry about.

It is harder and takes longer to wake from delta sleep than from any other sleep stage. But since what Tertullian accurately called "heavy sleep" and scientists now call "delta sleep" seldom occurs in the morning, you are unlikely to have any problems in arising from it at dawn.

If you take a morning snooze, you're apt to dream and awake from REM sleep. But if you nap in the afternoon, you're more likely to plummet into and arise from delta sleep. You'll tend to be more confused if aroused from a nap by a ringing telephone in the afternoon than in the morning. If disturbed from an afternoon "delta nap," you'll have difficulty picking up the phone and speaking coherently. Unless you explain, your caller might even think you're drunk. Moreover, if you plunge back to sleep, you're apt to forget, after rising again, that the conversation ever occurred. Therefore, if your afternoon shut-eye is disrupted by a telephone message, you may wish to write it down. (Because daytime naps, regardless of the hour, often interfere with nightly sleep, I hope you won't be napping at all.)

Chemicals, whether drugs or alcohol, also affect your manner of awakening. They make getting up more difficult, because they disrupt natural sleep. To aggravate matters, the sedative effects of alcohol and many drugs exert a direct influence on the brain's arousal apparatus. Consequently, the arduousness of climbing out of bed in the morning is compounded by "chemical sleep."

Hangovers

The most obvious problem for those waking up from "chemical sleep" is the *hangover*. The hangover is a way of life for some and a social institution for others. The first hangover is often viewed as a rite of passage for boys entering manhood. As feminist ideals flourish, this ridiculous custom will undoubtedly be accepted as a milestone on a girl's path toward womanhood. But after the hangover has served this symbolic function, it becomes a mere nuisance.

No physiological system escapes the influence of alcohol. Alcohol accelerates heart rate, dilates blood vessels to the brain, lowers blood sugar and body salt, and dehydrates your entire body, to mention only some of its effects. These actions culminate in throbbing morning-after headaches. Because changing positions aggravates the headache, you're inclined to remain immobilized in bed.

The extent to which alcohol produces a hangover is determined not only by what and how you drink, but also by your genetic makeup. For example, orientals have a low tolerance for alcohol and a high susceptibility to hangovers. Even within ethnic groups, individuals vary considerably in their physiological responses to alcohol. Whereas your neighbor might down a keg of beer and leap out of bed in the morning, you might be saddled with a hangover after nipping a mere bottle.

The best way to avoid a hangover is to drink moderately

and slowly. Don't imbibe on an empty stomach. Enjoy some food when you drink. Most important, know your limitations and stick to them.

Because of the way alcohol produces a hangover, the following measures are also worth remembering:

• *On arising with a hangover, consume several cups of well-salted beef or chicken broth*. Drinking only water will not help and may even increase nausea. Your body needs salt in order to retain water, water to compensate for dehydration, and rehydration to overcome a hangover. Salty broth should be taken hourly until the hangover disappears. If you anticipate a hangover, drink a salty broth before retiring; you may alleviate, if not prevent, the next morning's agony. If you're on a salt-restricted diet, check with your physician before you consume extra salt.

• *Eat or drink fructose*. By taking fructose, a type of sugar, you accomplish two things at once. Fructose supplies energy by replenishing the sugar lost from drinking. It also hastens the metabolic elimination of alcohol. Honey is loaded with fructose; fruits, vegetables, and vegetable extracts, especially tomato juice, are other excellent sources of fructose. A considerate host may add honey to his canapés. Toast dripping with honey is a simple but effective prebed remedy. During the hangover, tomato or mixed vegetable juices make a superb morning-after cocktail. (Avoid orange or other citric juices; they upset the stomach.)

• *Although you don't want to, get up anyway*. The main reason your head throbs is because the arteries leading to it are dilated. The faster they become constricted, the faster your hangover vanishes. And the quickest way to help narrow these vessels is to climb out of bed, move around, and apply ice packs to your head.

• *Above all else, don't try to alleviate your hangover with more alcohol*. Morning drinking will not quell, and may even aggravate, your hangover; it's also a sign of alcoholism. If you crave a cocktail on arising, make it a fruit or vegetable cocktail.

If alcohol and sleeping pills (hypnotics) are taken together, oversleeping is likely and an accidental suicide is possible. The tranquilizing power of a single sleeping pill can be magnified two to four times when consumed with alcohol. The notorious Mickey Finn is a combination of alcohol and the hypnotic chloral hydrate. Even when used without alcohol, sleeping pills can make it harder for you to drag yourself out of bed in the morning (Chapter 9).

Sleep Drunkenness

If you oversleep almost every day and are nearly impossible to arouse, you may unknowingly have a specific medical disorder called *sleep drunkenness*. People struck by this inelegantly named condition appear as if they had gotten thoroughly plastered the night before, even though they haven't touched a drop.

On getting up they are profoundly confused, disoriented, and uncoordinated for fifteen to sixty minutes, and often up to four hours. They rarely awake spontaneously, usually being oblivious to ringing clocks or telephones and even to repeating alarm clocks ("snooze alarms"). But if awakened, they'll quickly extinguish the alarm and promptly drop off again. When they finally arise, they may forget that they were awake before. By the time they gather their wits together, they're often late for work and, like Robert, eventually fired.

They sleep with a vengeance. Within two minutes, if not fifteen seconds, of going to bed, they're sound asleep. They describe their sleep as "extremely deep," like a general anesthesia. Although 75 percent of them have a normal distribution of nightly sleep stages (including REM), the majority deny ever dreaming. If they retire at nine in the evening, they may not awake on their own until one or two the following afternoon. Despite all this sleep, 88 percent of them are episodically drowsy throughout the day. This excessive daytime sleepiness, called *hypersomnia*, is discussed more thoroughly in Chapter 10. When hypersomnia accompanies sleep drunkenness, patients usually sleep an additional one to four hours during the day. At times they'll sleep for twenty-four hours straight.

Beside the obvious difficulties arising from inordinate sleepiness, some, although certainly not all, of these patients have other medical and psychiatric problems. Tension and migraine headaches are common. Depression, anxiety, rapid mood swings, and poor concentration may accompany sleep drunkenness. Nevertheless, many of these patients are totally free of these auxiliary symptoms. Contrary to some previous scientific reports—not to mention common sense—patients with sleep drunkenness do not have a characteristic personality type.

A third of them have been oversleeping since early childhood; the remainder started between the ages of eleven and thirty. It appears that once the symptoms begin, if unattended, they persist for life. Some patients report having hypersomnia with sleep drunkenness for over forty years. Men and women are affected equally, and slightly over a third of them having a close relative with the condition.

Contrary to what you might expect, these patients do not have a slow metabolism. Their heart and respiratory rates are actually higher than those of normal sleepers. If a sluggish metabolism is not the culprit, what is? Nobody knows.

The prevalence of this problem is also unknown. Except in extreme cases, it is hard to distinguish normally long sleepers from those afflicted with sleep drunkenness. This difficulty creates problems for researchers and patients. Zealous oversleepers often assume they simply need a lot of rest; they don't imagine they might have a specific medical disorder and hence are unlikely to seek professional help. Consequently, sleep experts have little way of knowing precisely how many people actually suffer from sleep drunkenness. As the public becomes increasingly aware of sleep disorders and clinics, however, researchers are discovering many new cases and are starting to believe that the problem is much more pervasive than was previously recognized.

If you suspect you may have sleep drunkenness, find out.

Because most physicians are still unfamiliar with sleep
drunkenness, consult, if possible, a sleep disorders clinic
(Appendix A).

Good treatment is available. Stimulant drugs, such as
amphetamines (Dexedrine), methylphenidate (Ritalin), and
phenmetrazine (Preludin), can significantly mitigate sleep
drunkenness. One of these medications taken at bedtime
will usually ameliorate the next morning's symptoms. If the
stimulant interferes with sleep, it can be used immediately
on awakening. A family member might have to administer
the drug. But under no circumstances should you ever
medicate yourself. Stimulant drugs are potentially dangerous! (See Chapter 9). *Only physicians who are especially
cognizant of both sleep disorders and the hazards of stimulants should prescribe them for you.*

Sleep drunkenness also puts a burden on family members.
Arousing the patient is a thankless task. The waker must be
vigorous and persistent. Because the oversleeper is irritable
and usually needs to be shaken repeatedly, he may become
physically abusive. After waking up, he may, if left alone,
quickly sneak back to sleep. Later he may feel guilty and
embarrassed for having been so petulant in the morning.
Despite all their efforts, the waker may feel unappreciated,
frustrated, and angry. Therefore, it's important that everybody in the family recognize that sleep drunkenness is a real
medical disorder and not mere laziness. If you live with
someone who suffers from sleep drunkenness, do not take
their morning obstreperousness personally. It's simply part
of the illness.

Whereas true sleep drunkenness is a chronic disorder
occurring almost every morning, perfectly healthy people
can occasionally fall victim to some of its symptoms.
Prolonged confusion and a stubborn urge to sleep may ensue
if you're suddenly awakened following too little sleep or
shortly after dozing off—especially in unfamiliar surroundings. A bout of sleep drunkenness can also happen when
you're unduly fatigued or run down or after you've consumed alcohol, hypnotics, or sedatives.

Oversleeping as an Escape

The prospect of a gloomy day can make staying in bed more appealing than leaving it. Indeed, studies reveal that people sleep longer when uninterested in their daily activities. On the other hand, you may be unaware, or at least understandably reluctant to admit, that your oversleeping is a refuge from a dreary job or an unsatisfying marriage. As I discuss in Chapter 10, certain types of depressed patients consistently oversleep. for some of you, rectifying life problems may be necessary if you're to awake on time.

I can't tell you how to alter an unhappy life. But I can suggest that while you're contemplating change you might arise sooner and easier, if you start the day with an activity sure to be pleasurable. You might routinely set aside thirty minutes after waking up to play with the kids, have breakfast with the family, or jog. By doing so, at least until other problems are resolved, you will have something immediately worthwhile to get up for.

Before jumping to the conclusion that your oversleeping is a retreat from life's disappointments, make sure that you read this entire chapter. Later on you'll see how disturbed circadian rhythms may be the hidden culprit for your difficulties in awakening. Although everybody can point to a distressing life problem, few people can spot a dysfunctional circadian rhythm. Consequently, you might incorrectly identify emotional factors rather than abnormal circadian rhythms as being responsible for your oversleeping. This is a vital distinction. In the former case, waking up more readily necessitates changing a part of your life; in the latter case, it requires altering the schedule of your life.

If you're inclined to impute psychological causes to physical problems, you should be especially cautious about assuming that your oversleeping is an emotional escape. Because everybody has complaints about spouse, job, or life, you can always identify some upsetting situation to account for your maladies. The mere existence of emotional predicaments does not mean they are necessarily responsible for oversleeping. After all, I don't know anybody who doesn't enjoy sleeping. Although he ruled most of Europe, Napoleon Bonaparte could say, "What a delightful thing rest is! The bed has become a place of luxury to me. I would not exchange it for all the thrones of the world."

To varying degrees, psychological retreats from the world and disturbances in circadian rhythm may both contribute to your oversleeping. As you will see, emotions influence circadian rhythms and vice versa. Consequently, pay attention to both potential causes.

How Not to Cope with Oversleeping

Misguided remedies abound. Just as "everybody" has the definitive nostrum for getting to sleep, "everybody" also has the surefire recipe for waking up.

Inclined to be a dragger myself, I've received a smorgasbord of suggestions. Wake up to music, not to an alarm. Place my clock in a barely reachable spot. Buy a "snooze alarm." Have my wife hide the clock in a different location every night so that I'm compelled to scurry around in the morning in order to extinguish it. Think positively about the day. Start arising by wiggling my toes, and gradually progress up my body, shaking every appendage with increasing vigor as I go along. (When I tried this, my wife had a fit, and I felt ridiculous feigning an epileptic seizure.) Spray water in my face. Wake to a strobe light, preferably accompanied by the "Anvil Chorus." Who knows? If a gimmick works, use it.

Even without such advice, in your quest to arise quickly and easily, you may be operating under several widely held yet false assumptions. Indeed, "commonsensical" remedies may backfire. For example, going to bed earlier creates problems in falling asleep and does not help you awake any easier.

Sleeping a few additional hours in the morning generates its own share of difficulties. You actually become *less* alert when you do get up. To test the hypothesis that excessive sleep produces grogginess, Dr. Ralph Berger had student volunteers try to distinguish split-second durations among a series of buzzing doorbells. This task, which measures alertness, was conducted thirty minutes after awakening. Berger compared how students performed after sleeping their normal eight hours with how they did if compelled to snooze for an extra three hours. The hypothesis was confirmed. After sleeping eleven hours, the students detected fewer long buzzes and mistook more short buzzes for long ones. This investigation, which has been replicated, indicates that additional sleep aggravates grogginess on awakening. Moreover, an extended morning catnap diminishes prior wakefulness, disrupts your sleep-wake cycle, and makes it harder to sleep that night. Thus, although catching a few extra winks in the morning is certainly tempting and seems like an obvious way to awake more refreshed, it actually leaves you less alert on arising and creates additional problems in getting to sleep.

For those of you whose predicament is the opposite of oversleeping—persistently waking up too early—forcing yourself to sleep longer in the morning will not help. You're probably trying to compel your body to sleep more than it needs to. If you wish to wake up later, go to bed later. When they go to bed sooner, older people frequently complain of awakening too early. Dr. Elliot Weitzman notes that many elderly patients consult him with the complaint "I can't stay asleep all night. I have to get up at 5 A.M. and by eight o'clock at night I'm terribly sleepy." consistently arising prematurely without being able to fall back to sleep might also be a sign of depression (Chapter 10).

A dreadful way to forestall morning fatigue and oversleeping, as opposed to sleep drunkenness, is to take stimulant drugs. Stimulants are also widely, albeit unwisely, used as an antidote for the daytime tiredness induced by hypnotics. Unless prescribed specifically for sleep drunkenness or narcolepsy (Chapter 10), as shown in Chapter 9, stimulants can often lead to drug dependency and sometimes to paranoia and psychosis.

On the other hand, over-the-counter, nonprescription "wake-up pills," such as NoDoz, are relatively harmless. Because the "magic" ingredient in most of these tablets is a hundred milligrams of caffeine, a cup of coffee will accomplish the same thing (Table 4.1). Though reasonably safe, caffeine is not innocuous. Before using it, review the section on caffeine in Chapter 4, especially the part that describes its adverse effects (pp. 66–68).

If your oversleeping is due to an altered circadian rhythm, caffeine will be of little help. Indeed, irregular biorhythms are a principal cause of waking-up difficulties.

The Rhythms of Life

A perplexed Charles Colton noted, "The bed is a bundle of paradoxes: we go to it with reluctance, yet we quit it with regret; we make up our minds every night to leave it early, but we make up our bodies every morning to keep it late."

Why this change of intentions? No single answer will suffice. Mere fickleness is too facile an explanation. But it's quite possible that these changing intentions partially stem from daily physiological alterations in our chemistry, mood, and behavior. Biologically speaking, the body you to go bed with is different from the one with which you arise. Perhaps these routine biological changes substantially account for Colton's paradox.

You have over a hundred different biological activities fluctuating in a regular daily pattern. For example, temperature, respiration, mood, alertness, and hormones each rise and fall at roughly the same time every day. These steady biological oscillations are called *circadian rhythms*. Coined by Dr. Franz Halberg, the term "circadian" derives from the Latin *circa* (around or about) and *dies* (day).

The duration of a biorhythmic* cycle varies, depending

---

*Preferring the more dignified term *chronobiology*, some scientists take offense at equating it with *biorhythms*, since the latter word suggests the often idiotic predictions found in newspapers. Nonetheless, although technically incorrect, I will employ the terms *biorhythms* and *chronobiology* synonymously—both meaning the objective quantification and investigation of timed biologic, and usually rhythmic, life functions.

on the particular biological function involved. Menstruation usually begins every thirty days. Already you've seen that during sleep REM-NREM cycles repeat every ninety minutes. The relative mental activity and quiescence of REM and NREM sleep respectively may even persist into wakefulness. If you pay close attention, you might notice your energy wax and wane throughout the day in a regular, possibly even a ninety-minute, pattern.

Most circadian rhythms, however, ebb and flow every twenty-five hours. Why these biorhythms fluctuate every twenty-five hours rather than every twenty-three or twenty-seven hours is unknown. But according to Dr. Weitzman, a major reason biological days differ slightly from solar days is that they allow people to adapt to different periods of light and dark with the changing seasons. There exist many examples of twenty-five-hour circadian rhythms. Stress hormones like cortisol normally reach their highest levels at 8 A.M. and dip to their lowest levels at midnight. With uncanny regularity, severely depressed patients are at their worst in the morning and gradually feel better as the day proceeds.

Although varying from person to person, body temperature rises during the day, usually peaking between noon and mid-afternoon. It then drops at night, bottoming out between midnight and 3 A.M. When your temperature is at its highest, you feel and function best; when your temperature is at its lowest, you feel and perform worst. It's no coincidence, therefore, that another twenty-five-hour circadian rhythm, the sleep-wake cycle, is synchronized with temperature fluctuations. When you're asleep, your temperature, alertness, mood, and physical proficiency are at their lowest; when you're fully awake, they're at their highest. The chill you may experience on waking in the middle of the night may be due as much to a low circadian temperature as to the cold weather or inadequate heating. Thus, your difficulty in functioning when you awake in the middle of the night may not only be due to sleeplessness, but also to the physiological activities influenced by your biological clock not performing at peak efficiency.

The timing of your circadian rhythms determines if you're a "lark" or an "owl." Larks are "day people." They are in high gear by dawn and fizzle out by dusk. Owls are "night people." They muddle through the morning, start to come alive by mid-afternoon, and are on full throttle by evening. These differences result from circadian rhythms. The temperature of a lark peaks in the morning and plummets at night. On the other hand, the temperature of an owl drops in the morning and rises later on.

Although biologically endowed, circadian rhythms can be altered slightly by the environment. Otherwise, how could twenty-five-hour circadian functions accommodate to the twenty-four-hour days imposed on us by the sun?

Zeitgebers (i.e., indicators of time) synchronize this adjustment by serving as relatively consistent temporal reference points. Zeitgebers include clocks, regularly timed meals and television programs, work shifts, the amount of darkness outdoors, and the sun's position in the sky. If they occur at roughly the same time every day, zeitgebers help to structure your biorhythms so that they conform to the demands of a twenty-four-hour day. By doing so, zeitgebers compress biological clocks to adjust to societal clocks.

When not enough zeitgebers are available to shape biorhythmic patterns, circadian rhythms float aimlessly. In the absence of well-structured circadian patterns, biological clocks become desynchronized. For example, whereas on awakening your temperature and other circadian functions are normally rising, when your biorhythms are disrupted and falling, your ability to perform effectively is impaired. So while your job is prompting you to wake up, your body is urging you to stay in bed.

Because circadian temperature fluctuations correlate with and affect *when* you are asleep and awake, measuring each of these factors provides valuable clues as to why you're having trouble getting up or falling asleep. To determine if desynchronized circadian rhythms are responsible for your waking and sleeping difficulties, record three items: (a) the approximate time you fall asleep, (b) the time you awake, and (c) your temperature several times throughout the day.

To enhance accuracy and to see your overall circadian pattern, record all these items for any convenient but *consecutive* four to five days. When doing so, follow your typical sleeping and waking habits.

Take your temperature four times daily: on arising, on retiring, and at two other evenly spaced times during the day (e.g., noon and 6 P.M.). Because your temperature may vary by only a degree or so throughout the day, it's essential to make accurate thermometer readings. Do not eat not drink just before taking your temperature. Leave the thermometer under your tongue for a full four minutes. If you're ill, even if you *don't* have a fever, hold off taking your temperature. Menstruation may also affect them. Therefore, don't measure your temperature five days before and during menstrual periods.

When monitoring your temperature as well as your sleep and wake times for four or five consecutive days, make a graph of Figure 8.1, using the format illustrated in Figures 8.2A and 8.2B.

Figure 8.2A shows typical temperature fluctuations and their usual relationships to normal sleep-wake cycles. Figure 8.2B depicts temperature oscillations that are out of kilter with sleeping and waking.

After graphing your own findings on Figure 8.1, you'll be prepared to determine if circadian disturbances are contributing to your waking and sleeping problems. The sooner you begin your recordings, the sooner you'll be able to get the answers—so start today!

Coping with Biorhythm Difficulties

Your circadian graph may uncover a biorhythmic predicament. As Figure 8.2A illustrates, temperature is normally low during sleeping hours and high during the peak waking hours. If your graph resembles this pattern, it's unlikely that circadian-rhythm disturbances account for your problem. But if your temperature is relatively high on going to bed, you may have trouble falling asleep. If your temperature is

FIGURE 8.1
YOUR CIRCADIAN-RHYTHM CHART

Record the times at which you fell asleep, awoke, and took your temperature.

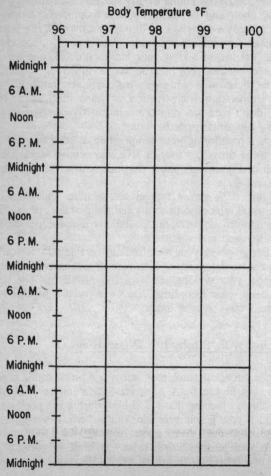

Body Temperature °F

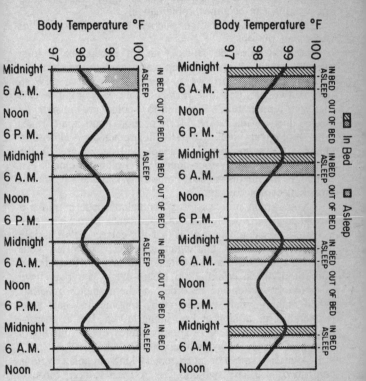

FIGURE 8.2A
SYNCHRONIZED
CIRCADIAN RHYTHM

FIGURE 8.2B
DESYNCHRONIZED
CIRCADIAN RHYTHM

Above left: Note how temperature peaks at about the same time every day. Also observe that temperature is at its lowest during sleep and at its highest in the afternoon.

Above right: Although this is a predictable circadian pattern, the highest temperature occurs at midnight, making it difficult to fall asleep. Daytime fatigue and poor performance are likely to exist when daytime temperature is relatively low.

relatively low or declining when you want to get up, you're likely to oversleep, or at least to have a difficult time waking up. Thus, when temperature fluctuations fail to harmonize with your desired sleep schedule, as in Figure 8.2B, sleeping and waking can become problematical.

Desynchronized circadian sleep-wake patterns occur for two major reasons.

First, you may be stuck with an exceptionally long circadian cycle. A normal sleep-wake-temperature circadian cycle is completed in twenty-five hours, give or take an hour or two. It's possible, however, that your graph reveals that your temperature's high and low points are *consistently* spaced thirty or maybe even forty or more hours apart. If so, your biological clock, even with tremendous efforts to change it, cannot possibly adapt with any ease to the demands of a twenty-four-hour day. Biological clocks can be nudged but not dismantled. Fortunately, extremely protracted circadian cycles are rare.

If your graph indicates this anomalous pattern, make a second graph with newly taken measurements. Before accepting a distressing diagnosis, check that it's correct. It's possible that a subtle illness that went undetected distorted your initial graph. You may have taken medication that altered your biorhythms. Waking up bleary-eyed, you may have inaccurately gotten or recorded a thermometer reading. When making your second graph, continue to chart your temperature on arising and on going to bed. But to guarantee greater accuracy, record temperatures every four hours (instead of twice a day) while you're awake.

If your assessment of an extremely long circadian cycle is confirmed, you have two choices. You can struggle through as you now do, but at least knowing why your alertness and performance levels rise and fall at peculiar times. Armed with this information, you can try, when possible, to plan around your "bioarrhythmias." Some of the tricks and troubles in doing so are discussed in the next two sections on "Shift Workers" and "Jet Lag."

Your second option is to substantially, if not radically, alter your life style. Before you take this plunge, however, it's vital that you have your diagnosis corroborated by the staff of a sleep disorders clinic (Appendix A). If you obtain a professional confirmation, you might wish to rearrange your work schedule so that it's in greater harmony with your prolonged circadian pattern. Your boss, however, may look at you cross-eyed if you merely state your predicament. Claiming you have an incredibly long circadian rhythm that necessitates an altered work schedule sounds fishy at best. A doctor's letter from the sleep disorders clinic, validating the diagnosis and explaining its implications, may go a long way to reducing your boss's understandable skepticism. After all, if adjusting your work schedule allows you to produce at peak efficiency, both you *and* your employer benefit.

It's quite possible that your line of work does not allow for such flexibility. Changing occupations may be the only way out of your dilemma. An advertising executive with literary aspirations may wish to become a free-lance writer. A hospital nurse on a fixed morning shift may want to work independently as a private-duty nurse to suit her own biorhythmic pattern. Once you know when you can or cannot function at your best, you can plan your schedule accordingly.

Inadequate or constantly shifting zeitgebers give rise to the other major (and more common) cause for desynchronized circadian rhythms. Routinely living by zeitgebers, those indicators of time, is necessary for structuring *regular* circadian patterns. Normally, temperature, wakefulness, and performance levels peak concurrently because you train them to do so by following a standard routine. You wake, eat, work, and retire at roughly the same time every day.

By persistently waking at different times, however, your biorhythms are denied the opportunity to settle into a fixed schedule. If you arise one day at 9 A.M., the next day at 2 P.M., and the one after that at 7 A.M., how can your body "know" which circadian rhythm to establish? Should it "plan" a day starting at 7 A.M., 9 A.M., or 2 P.M.? Similarly, if your major productivity occurs in the morning one day and late at night on the next, your body becomes "confused"; it can't "figure out" when you want your biorhythms to rise and fall.

By not sticking to a regular schedule, the self-employed, unemployed, and socially isolated are most likely to have circadian-rhythm disturbances. Most successful authors, even if they're free-lancing, adhere to a fixed schedule. Steady work habits not only give rise to achievement through "discipline" but also make this achievement possible by maintaining regular circadian rhythms.

If your temperature graph reveals an irregular circadian pattern, you should, in order to wake (or fall asleep) comfortably, try to standardize your biorhythms. Because you can force wakefulness, but not sleep, you can properly synchronize your biorhythms by adopting these five rules:

1. *Eliminate all naps.*
2. *Go to bed only when you're sleepy.*
3. *Wake up at the same time every day—including weekends.* Avoid the temptation to catch a few extra winks on your days off. It requires a minimum of several weeks to reestablish a regular circadian pattern. Interrupting your attempts on weekends will vitiate all of your prior efforts during the week, and you'll have to start all over again. (Moreover, there's no point to oversleeping; as noted before, it only fosters additional grogginess when you do awake.)
4. *Schedule your most productive hours for the same time every day.* If during the week you work from 9 A.M. to 5 P.M., on Saturdays and Sundays perform activities requiring energy and alertness from roughly 9 A.M. to 5 P.M. Whether you're cleaning the house, fixing a bicycle, playing football, or studying physics, keep training your circadian rhythms on weekends.
5. *Establish a daily routine.* Without making a pest of yourself, try when possible to eat, relax, and do other things at approximately the same time every day. But don't get carried away! It is unnecessary and downright crazy to do exactly the same thing every hour of every day. To synchronize your circadian rhythms, you need only establish a few daytime zeitgebers, or points of reference. For example, in

addition to following the preceding four rules, having three meals at about the same time every day, including weekends, will suffice.

Don't expect overnight results. Don't even expect to adopt all of these measures at once. The longer you've had problems waking and sleeping, the longer it takes to correct irregular circadian rhythms. If your troubles have existed for only several months, you will have to adhere to these rules for two to three weeks before your biorhythms become fully harmonized. But if you've been plagued for years, progress will take considerably longer. Realistically speaking, you will not be able to follow all five rules immediately; you'll have to proceed gradually.

Although Amy was never a good sleeper, her difficulties really started when she was thrown by a runaway horse. Because her mishap resulted in a severe fracture followed by medical complications, Amy had to spend five months at home before her leg had fully healed. Unable to return to college and having nothing else to do, she listlessly passed the days playing records, watching television, and seeing an occasional visitor. Her days and nights blended, neither one having any particular purpose. She slept at will. When her leg was finally mended, she was sleeping fitfully for twelve hours a day. On returning to college, she felt perpetually tired. "Getting to sleep took forever and getting up took even longer." During the ensuing nine years, she married happily, abused hypnotics periodically, and slept erratically.

When we first met, Amy napped four to six hours a day, slept three hours a night, and was exhausted the rest of the time. About once a week she spent a whole day lying in bed. Even though she was healthy in every other respect, she was as crippled as she had been right after being thrown by that horse. Her temperature graph revealed an erratic circadian pattern. Fortunately, Amy was no longer using sleeping pills; otherwise her recovery would have taken several additional months, because of the need to withdraw her from hypnotics.

Though eagerly wanting help, she was unable to adopt

the five rules immediately. Instead, we agreed that she would try to move gradually toward following these rules. Each month Amy napped one hour less a day. Whereas before she used to lie in bed at least till noon, she now started waking up half an hour earlier each month. Initially, she arose at 11:30 A.M., a month later at 11:00 A.M., and so forth, until she reached 9:00 A.M. Adhering to a regular schedule, Amy slowly increased her daytime activities. At the beginning she made it her business to shop, clean, pick up her daughters, or run errands from 2 P.M. to 5 P.M. Four months later she was sufficiently awake and alert in the afternoon to work as a part-time college research assistant.

A year after her first consultation, Amy usually awoke at 9 A.M., worked regularly, and experienced a new vitality. She continued to nap around 6 P.M., and took over an hour to fall asleep at night. Nevertheless, the tenacity with which she gradually formed a regular circadian rhythm paid off. If Amy had attempted to follow all the rules at once, she probably would have failed and retreated to bed. But by making stepwise changes, and by recording her temperature chart monthly to see tangible evidence of an emerging circadian pattern, she was sufficiently encouraged to persist.

Although I moved to another city, we've exchanged Christmas cards for the past six years. Her last card read in part, "If there ever was a 'sandwoman,' . . . I was her. I'm still dragging my tail by dinner time and take about twenty minutes to crawl out of bed. But my days belong to me. . . . You'd be proud of me—hell, I'm proud of me!"

Amy's problem was protracted and severe; she *had* to proceed gradually. How quickly you should proceed depends on your "will power" and on how long your difficulties have existed.

If waking up has been a struggle for *over* a year, map out a reasonable timetable for adopting these rules. Knowing yourself best, you should decide to take a new step every week, every two weeks, or whenever. Just make sure that you're moving toward a goal, and don't be upset by momentary setbacks; everybody has them. Despite all of her determination, Amy occasionally overslept during the initial months of her recovery. But her fortitude, combined with her family's support, enabled her to continue relatively unfazed by these periodic lapses.

If your problems of waking have occurred for *less* than a year, try adopting these rules all at once. If you can follow them, great. If not, don't despair—just set up a stepwise program.

Don't worry—you will *not* have to adhere to these rules forever. When you are waking with relative comfort, you can occasionally depart from these guidelines without adverse consequences. After all, occasionally irregular schedules are regular parts of life. It is when these exceptions become routine that sleeping and waking become troublesome. Indeed, because of twentieth-century technological innovations, these constant changes of routine have created new sleeping and waking dilemmas for millions.

Shift Workers

Thomas Edison felt that sleep was a self-indulgent waste of time and hoped that his electric light bulb would all but eliminate the need for it. His invention did affect sleep, but not in the way he intended. Electric lighting, along with indoor heating, telephones, and most recently computers, have transformed social productivity from a "nine-to-five" to a twenty-four-hours-a-day endeavor. Greater industrial competition and the need to offer more jobs and goods to an expanding populace have led many factories to operate around the clock. Day and night, we expect law enforcement, fire protection, medical care, sanitation, transportation, and communication. If the grocery and the drug store are open *all* the time, so much the better. Unfortunately, technological progress and social advances have outstripped biological adaptation.

A twenty-four-hour economy has generated an accelerating number of "off-hour" or shift workers with circadian rhythm problems. As of May, 1977, about 9 percent of Americans employed full-time (excluding farmers) regularly

worked between 4 P.M. and midnight, whereas 4 percent
worked between midnight and 8 A.M. Men compose 62, 67,
and 75 percent of the labor force on days, evenings, and
nights, respectively. Approximately 70 percent of all men
and half of all women who are off-hour shift workers are
married. Wishing to be with their families and participate in
the daytime world, many shift workers prefer rotating between days and nights. If you're a rotating-shift workers,
these constant changes disrupt and prevent you from
establishing a firm circadian rhythm. Just when your daytime circadian pattern is formed, you move onto the evening
or the night shift, and by the time a new biorhythmic pattern
is established, you're back on the day shift.

Ominous difficulties can result from these desynchronized
circadian patterns. For example, hospital interns must help
patients in the middle of the night when their alertness and
efficiency are most impaired. Add to this the effects of sleep
deprivation, and you are left with a sobering, if not terrifying scenario. If you're sufficiently ill to require a physician
at 3 A.M., your need is at its highest just when the doctor's
proficiency is at its lowest.

Circadian-rhythm disturbances afflict shift workers in every industry. Night workers produce less and cause more
errors than their daytime counterparts. Gastrointestinal symptoms (e.g., poor appetite, stomach upsets, nausea, diarrhea,
constipation) plague 25 to 50 percent of all shift workers.
According to one survey of male workers, complaints of
on-the-job fatigue came from 83 percent of the nighttime but from only 4 percent of daytime employees. At least
two studies specify sleep as *the* main problem of both male
and female shift workers.

If you are a shift worker, even the sleep you do manage
to obtain is unsatisfying. If you're working nights and go to
bed at 8 A.M., you'll have more REM, more brief awakenings, and a shorter sleep duration than nocturnal sleepers.

Night work does have its advantages—incentive pay and
compensatory time off. Many industries attempt to provide
increased quality control and safety standards during "off"
shifts. But these are social, not biological solutions.

There is, however, a simple and effective *biological* remedy. By working only nights, you will develop a well-formed circadian rhythm. Although biologically desirable, this solution is socially impractical. On your days off you'll want to join the daytime world. But your established nocturnal circadian pattern is not equipped to do so. If you grit your teeth and try to muddle through, your "old" (nighttime) biorhythm disintegrates; when you return to your usual night schedule, your circadian rhythm is once again impaired. A British survey demonstrated that only 25 percent of the workers adjusted to the night shift within five days. Many required two weeks, and some were unable to adapt at all.

These constant shift changes affect not only workers, but also their families. While one parent is working, the other is sleeping. Couples are denied normal companionship, increasing the chances for marital strife and divorce. Whereas the proportion of employees who are separated and divorced is only slightly higher among male off-hour workers, it is substantially higher among women; 21, 25, and 31 percent of day-, evening-, and night-working women respectively are separated or divorced. It is unknown whether separation and divorce led women to work late shifts, or whether working late shifts reflected or contributed to the dissolution of their marriages. It's unlikely, however, that working evenings, and especially nights, promotes family cohesiveness.

Children grow up essentially without one of their parents. Youngsters may wonder why their mom or dad does not play with them nearly as much as do their friends' parents. Because preschoolers may fail to understand why the working parent rarely sees them, they'll frequently blame themselves. The irrationality of childhood thinking may lead them to believe, "I must be bad, otherwise daddy would spend more time with me." It's important for the seven million American late-shift workers and their roughly seventeen million family members to appreciate and respond appropriately to these stresses.

There's no good solution to this problem. From a strictly biological perspective, alternating between days and nights every two weeks is sheer folly. Consistent night work obviates the biological difficulty, but it wipes out any remnants of a social life.

Out of this gloomy portrayal of the late-shift worker's dilemma comes one reassuring note. If, as an off-shift worker, you and your family understand that desynchronized circadian rhythms are substantially responsible for moodiness and problems in working, playing, sleeping, and waking, at least the mystery behind these difficulties is removed and a more sympathetic appreciation of what you're going through can emerge.

Jet Lag

Like the shift worker who moves from days to nights, the overseas traveler tries unsuccessfully to accommodate old biorhythms to new circumstances. Whereas changing time slots creates chronic distress for the shift worker, changing time zones creates merely transitory discomfort for the traveler. Moreover, the traveler's new environment "supports" his attempts to form a new circadian pattern. The late-shift worker is less fortunate; he and his body "know" that they are out of harmony with the dominant daytime society. Although less severe, jet lag plagues an ever-growing number of people as transoceanic travel increases.

If you leave New York at 10 P.M. and fly six hours to London, your "body time" on arrival is 4 A.M., while British time is 10 A.M. Although sleeping aboard your flight minimizes sleep loss, your circadian-rhythm problems remain. Because on your arrival your biological clock is set at 4 A.M., you're operating at minimum proficiency. At this juncture you face two less than satisfactory options. You can follow your "old" (New York) biorhythm by grabbing a snooze and waking up to a London afternoon. But by "easing" into the new situation in this way, you "lose" half a day, and will not fall asleep until way past midnight. Or, you can force yourself to stay awake in order to quickly establish a "new" (London) biorhythm. Because you're still functioning under your old circadian pattern, you're apt to stumble through the day, dine early, and retire by 9 P.M., which is 3 P.M. New York time. If on the day of your flight you arose at 9 A.M., that means you've been awake for thirty consecutive hours. Though you'll drop off in an instant, you'll probably get up at around 6 A.M. London time and twiddle your thumbs until the rest of London awakes. When you "ease" into the new environment, jet lag usually persists for two to four days. By staying awake after your arrival, you normally experience jet-lag fatigue for one or two days.

The duration and severity of jet lag vary according to other factors. Jet-lag distress increases with the number of hours flown and the number of time zones passed. Whether you fly east or west* is less important than when you arrive and for how long you stay. If instead you leave New York at 10 A.M. and arrive in London at 10 P.M. (4 P.M. in New York), by the time you pass through customs, dine, and check into your hotel, it will be about 2 A.M. at the earliest before you can go to bed. Although probably too early for you to fall asleep easily, considering that your "body time" is 8 P.M. and you've been awake for only about twelve hours, your circadian rhythm is almost in step with London time. If you're planning to stay abroad for more than a week, arriving at night and quickly establishing a new biorhythm is advantageous. But if you're to return in a day or two, you might as well stick to your old pattern; otherwise, when you arrive back home, your circadian difficulties will erupt all over again.

Although everybody is influenced by jet lag in a different way, nobody escapes it completely. If you arrive in London at 10 A.M. and feel fully confident that you can easily rush around without taking a nap, beware. Even if you are relatively immune to jet lag, don't forget that it still affects you. Being on vacation in a new place may cause you to

---

*Jet lag occurs only if you travel east or west; it does not develop if you go north or south. After you cross five time zones, the restoration of synchronized sleep-wake cycles typically requires two days when flying west and four days when flying east.

overlook that your circadian rhythm is at low ebb. Be extra careful crossing streets, because your alertness *will* be impaired, even if you're unaware of it. For this reason, many businessmen are forbidden, if flying over more than four time zones, to make significant corporate decisions for at least twenty-four hours. In *White House Years*, Henry Kissinger admits that on two separate occasions even he "paid a psychological price" by losing his temper at the secret Vietnam peace negotiations, because he attended them immediately after a long plane flight. If circumstances demand immediate decisions, executives and diplomats will schedule meetings so that they coincide with their old biorhythms. Airline officials claim that their crews are given enough time between flights to establish a new and stable circadian pattern, so as not to endanger their passengers.

Dr. C. C. Gullett, the corporate director of medical services for TWA, offers the following recommendations for overseas travelers: "Start in a rested state, avoid overindulgence of food and liquor enroute, rest or sleep when sleepy, (and) eat lightly to fit the appetite rather than the time of the day."

Until scientists discover ways to obviate biorhythmic problems, jet lag difficulties will persist. Circadian patterns are so ingrained in our species and in many others that even migrating birds pause when crossing more than four time zones.

Perhaps it's just as well that circadian disturbances exist. They act as vital, though discomfiting reminders that we pay a real price when technological progress exceeds our biological capabilities. The proliferation of drugs—another product of advancing technology—underscores this warning. The next chapter, which examines the effects of drugs on waking and sleeping, elaborates on this concern.

CHAPTER NINE

Breaking the Pill Habit

"It started so innocently," he mumbled. "It" was addiction to sleeping pills; "he" was Howard, a sixty-year-old lying helplessly in a hospital bed, both legs wrapped in gauze. This chimerical apparition—half mummy, half human—lost its mythical appearance quickly; for as I approached him, he became quite real. His extensive burns were not fully hidden by the bandages. Neither was his discomfort.

"Four years ago, my wife, Toby, got breast cancer and died five months later. It was horrible. We had been very close; friends called us the happiest couple they knew. During her last months we spent most of our time together. Toby rarely admitted it, but she was in constant pain. Although her doctor and I did everything possible to soothe it, nothing helped. The more I tried to cheer her up, the sadder I became. During Toby's last two months, she was in so much agony that two or three sleeping pills were necessary to get her to sleep. I put on a strong facade, but I too was crumbling inside and unable to sleep. Despite abhorring any kind of pills, I felt that unless I got some rest, I wouldn't be of *any* use to myself or to her. So like a kid sneaking behind the garage to puff a cigarette, I stole one of her sleeping pills. And for the first time in weeks, I slept through the night. That Nembutal* worked like magic; I was asleep in a flash and felt great in the morning. However, knowing the pills were dangerous, I resolved never to take another one.

"Then Toby died. I barely remember the next few weeks. I know I didn't sleep very well during that time, but that was natural, and furthermore I didn't care. Whereas before her illness, I would be asleep by eleven, now I couldn't fall asleep until two or three in the morning. I'd wake up several times during the night and end up waiting for dawn to appear. When it did, I'd crawl out of bed feeling as empty as our apartment seemed without her.

"After six weeks or so, I became restless and knew it was time to return to work. I did, but it wasn't the same. Until then my partner, Ben, and I had successfully run a dry-cleaning store. I had always liked talking with the customers and even keeping after the lousy help. But now everything was an effort; for the first time in twenty-three years I didn't care if the damn shirts were ready on time or if the presses were operating properly. I don't really know if this was mainly due to mourning or simply exhaustion, but in either case, I was making a mess of things. After I misplaced three orders one day, Ben finally blew his stack. I couldn't blame him. He'd been carrying the load all by himself for a long time. When he settled down, he told me to go home and get a good night's sleep. I agreed. After all, I figured, life must go on.

"That night I took one of Toby's Nembutals, and again slept like a log. The next day I awoke feeling that I could rejoin the living. Ben was thrilled and later me surprised me with tickets for that evening's hockey game; I'd always been a hockey nut. When I got home after the game, I was so excited, I couldn't fall asleep. Although tempted to take a Nembutal, I didn't. I only slept for a couple hours that night, but that was okay—I was turning the corner of my depression.

*Nembutal is a barbiturate used for calming the nerves and for inducing sleep. It belongs to a group of drugs called "hypno-sedatives."

"The next day, however, was a real grind. Having had only two or three hours of sleep, I was drained by mid-afternoon. Since I desperately wanted to get back into the swing of things, I *had* to sleep. For the next several nights I took Toby's Nembutal and slept peacefully.

"But when the weekend arrived and because the store was going to be closed, I didn't take a pill. I was still leery about becoming hooked. I remember thinking that only bums, junkies, and fools get addicted to sleeping pills. To my relief, that night I slept without difficulty. The following evening I also went to bed without a pill and quickly dropped off. About thirty minutes later, however, I awoke from the first of many nightmares. They were always the same. Toby was lying all disfigured in a block of ice that was being transported by a conveyer belt into a gigantic refrigerator. These dreams kept me drifting in and out of sleep the entire night.

"On Sunday night, even though I was tired, I just couldn't get to sleep. At about one in the morning I gave in and took a Nembutal. I reasoned, 'One little yellow capsule can't hurt. I'm intelligent and won't overdo it. Just when I'm rejoining the human race, I'm not going to let a dumb thing like insomnia get in my way.' I took a pill every night that week and slept wonderfully.

"Indeed, life *was* picking up for me. I was pulling more than my fair share at work. Ben took a well-deserved two-week vacation and I managed the store single-handedly. I hadn't felt that good for years.

"When Toby's Nembutal ran out, I easily got a prescription from my doctor. He glibly warned me about abusing pills, but I assured him that I rarely used them. It wasn't like me to lie, but it was only a tiny lie, and I didn't want to bother him with the whole story. Furthermore, once or twice a week I would go without taking a pill, and therefore I convinced myself I wasn't hooked.

"But after a month of using Nembutal almost every night, I began to have more difficulties sleeping. It would take me over an hour to drop off, and then, a whole series of frightening dreams would awake me several times a night. I

164	Jerrold S. Maxmen, M.D.

would get up at five and couldn't get back to sleep. I really wanted to enjoy work, but I was functioning at a snail's pace. In one day I made a $300 error adding receipts and forgot to lock the back door. I just wasn't paying attention; I was simply too exhausted.

"Then two punks held up the store. That night I needed, or maybe I felt entitled, to take two capsules. Regardless, I slept soundly.

"After a month, two pills were not enough. Even if I fell asleep, I'd soon wake up and spend the rest of the night fussing about not sleeping. I became increasingly irritated, and to calm my nerves I took a shot of whiskey. I hardly ever touched the stuff, but it *did* help me sleep.

"To make a long story short, over the next year I gradually took three, four, and then five pills to overcome insomnia.

"I knew I was hooked, but what could I do? I didn't want to tell my doctor; he might stop my pills. I was amazed that he hadn't already. I had to work, and to do that, I had to sleep. So I decided to wait for the weekend, and then to go 'cold turkey.' It was hell! I was completely drained, partially from sleeplessness, but also from a strange, creepy restlessness that kept getting worse. To stop me from jumping out of my skin, by Sunday night I capitulated and gobbled down a couple of Nembutal. It was like magic; in an hour I was relaxed and by the next day I was back, or almost back, to normal. Setting four capsules a night as my limit, when I later on had trouble sleeping, a shot of whiskey would always do the trick.

"Two weeks ago I went to the wedding of Ben's youngest son. I probably drank too much, but not *that* much—four or five at the most. I had a fabulous time: danced like Fred Astaire, even flirted a bit. When I finally got home, I took my usual four Nembutal along with a nightcap. But I still couldn't drop off. So I lay in bed, watched a late movie, and smoked a cigarette.

"Things become hazy at this point. I know I couldn't sleep and that I had an especially busy day tomorrow because the inventory had to be completed. I took several more drinks and a couple more pills. At the time I couldn't remember exactly how many Nembutal I'd used, and that it didn't really matter since I felt immune to the stuff. After that, everything's a blank. Evidently, I fell asleep, my cigarette started a fire, and my apartment went up in flames. I understand that a fireman rescued me just in time to save my life, or what's left of it.

"The next thing I remember is waking up in the burn unit. Because the doctors were so worried that I'd die, and I was not thinking very clearly, nobody knew I had been using Nembutal. A couple days later that eery, restless feeling returned, but I blamed it on my burns and my being confined to bed. Then, a week after I was admitted, I reportedly had a convulsion. I don't remember that either. The doctors tell me the seizure was caused by my withdrawing from too much booze and pills.

"So here I am. My legs itch all over, my skin—or what's left of it—hurts like hell, my sleep is lousy, my mind's in a fog, my apartment is ruined, and the doctors don't even know when I'll be discharged. Remember I told you that only bums, junkies, and fools get addicted. I must be all three."

With the help of two skin grafts and special medical and nursing care over the next five months, Howard's burns healed and he was withdrawn safely from Nembutal at the rate of one capsule every two weeks. After his pills were stopped, he continued to have problems sleeping for nearly a year. Progressive relaxation and soporific phrases helped, but the deeper physical and emotional scars remained. His body had been so acclimated to Nembutal that it was difficult for Howard to concentrate and function effectively in a non-drugged condition. Despite everything that had happened and even though he resisted, he still craved Nembutal. "It's spooky. I know that I can't touch the stuff, but whenever I think about sleep, which is most of the time, I'm tempted to take a Nembutal. It's like Faust is hiding inside that yellow capsule. I often feel it's the only thing that could *totally* put me at ease. And that scares me!"

It's been two years since the fire, and Howard has retired

to Arizona. Despite an occasional restless night, he's learned to sleep soundly and live comfortably without pills and alcohol.

"But I'm Not Like Howard"

If Howard's experience with Nembutal, a barbiturate hypno-sedative, seems extraordinary, let me assure you it isn't. If you still think his saga is uncommonly grotesque, keep in mind these conservative estimates for 1976:

- Some 9,000,000 Americans used hypnotics.
- Hypno-sedatives were found in the bloodstreams of 11 percent of the drivers and 5 percent of the pedestrians who were killed in traffic accidents.
- About 40,400 people were treated for primary* hypno-sedative use.
- An additional 32,000 people were being treated for secondary* hypno-sedative abuse.
- Barbiturates are the most frequently used drugs for suicide, accounting for 30 percent of the 7,500 deaths from intentional overdosing.
- Over 2,300 deaths resulted from accidental hypno-sedative overdoses.
- Hypno-sedatives were taken for roughly 500,000 attempted suicides.

These figures would be even more alarming if they included other medications often used to induce sleep, such as over-the-counter sleep aids, antidepressants, major tranquilizers, and opiates. Add to this list the *most* widely employed soporific agent, alcohol, and you can magnify all of these figures threefold or even fivefold!

*Because sleeping-pill addicts frequently use several drugs at once, "primary" hypno-sedative abuse refers to the case in which hypno-sedative habituation is the main problem. "Secondary" hypno-sedative abuse means that although hypno-sedatives were being taken, the misuse of other drugs was the chief object of treatment.

A problem with statistics like these is that once the figures become so large, they're "just" big numbers. In a sense, whether 300,000 or 700,000 people attempted suicide with hypno-sedatives doesn't matter. Either statistic is overwhelming and tragic.

Statistics are impersonal. They indicate the scope but not the soul of a problem. They don't reflect the frustration of sleepless nights, the agony of being perpetually fatigued and numbed, the helplessness of trying to break the sleeping-pill habit, the loss of productivity and pride, the sorrow of loved ones, or the nagging fear that you're killing yourself.

If these concerns strike you as melodramatic and not applicable to you, think again. At the beginning Howard exercised caution; he knew that sleeping pills were dangerous. But like many people who misuse hypnotics, Howard started to take pills during periods of stress. When these stresses passed, however, his Nembutal dependence had already developed a "life of its own." For a long time Howard didn't believe the pills controlled him. Hypnotic addiction evolves like alcoholism. There is a Japanese proverb that goes, "First the man takes a drink, then the drink takes a drink, then the drink takes the man." Howard deceived himself into thinking that *only* "the other guy" is stupid enough or lacks the self-control to get hooked.

Howard's downfall was not due to a lack of knowledge or even to Nembutal; it was caused by *self-deception*. Whenever he "had" to sleep, he always could find a "justifiable" reason for taking a pill. He needed to help his dying wife. He needed to function at work. He needed an extra pill because he was upset by having been robbed. He needed a Nembutal to "rejoin the human race." All these excuses are perfectly understandable, given his difficult circumstances. Almost anybody would be tempted to resort to a "harmless" sleeping pill during miserable times. But it is just because anybody might do so under trying conditions that the potential for self-deception is so great, and the insidious development of hypnotic abuse so enormous. In the midst of a real crisis, you may naturally seek immediate comfort in a pill and not worry about long-range, seemingly hypothetical consequences.

Although the details of Howard's story are unique, we can all deceive ourselves into hypnotic abuse. You may have different problems, you may suffer to a different extent, you may use hypnotics in different ways, and you may deceive yourself by different means. But we *all* possess psychologies and physiologies that respond to hypnotics in many *identical* ways. That is why it is vital to understand how sleeping pills can affect you. But as important as it is to learn all the "facts," knowing them is useless if you con yourself into believing that they don't apply to *you*.

It's Your Choice

If you're taking sleeping pills, stop. If you're not, don't start.

This is basically sound advice. Hypnotics disrupt sleep and induce fatigue. Sleeping pills are dangerous; using them can lead to addiction and death. The scientific verdict on sleeping pills is clear—they're a menace.

It is with great reluctance, therefore, that I say that, *under very special circumstances,* sleeping pills can be helpful and safe. Many experts will dispute this statement. They will understandably claim that sleeping pills should never be used. I disagree.

I am *not* advocating the use of hypnotics The previous chapters have presented many effective and, in my opinion, preferable methods of falling and staying asleep. I say, "in my opinion" because my favoring "natural" ways of fostering sleep, although based principally on scientific evidence, is also influenced by personal experience. I've just seen too many Howards, too many good people's lives, devastated by sleeping pills to feel otherwise. But I also know a great many who properly and occasionally use sleeping pills. Nothing dreadful happens to them. To ignore that sleeping pills are sometimes helpful is to ignore reality.

The debate over whether sleeping pills should ever be

taken is so clouded by rhetoric that people wishing to learn the real facts are apt to suspect anything they hear. It may well be that drug companies make 100 million to 175 million dollars annually by selling hypnotics, that Americans consume over three billion doses of sleeping pills weighing 600 tons a year, that doctors unnecessarily write 25 million prescriptions for sleeping pills a year, that pharmaceutical houses annually produce enough hypnotics to put every American to sleep for 200 hours, and that we are a "drugged society." But we are also a free society. If provided with honest and complete information, people will, let us hope, make intelligent choices about the drugs they take. Even if justified, tirades against avaricious drug companies, stupid doctors, and moral decay have no bearing on whether you in particular will be helped or harmed by sleeping pills.

I want to give you this information and allow you to make up your own mind. Although I would much prefer that you abstain from using any sleeping pills, if you choose to do so, I would like you to know how they are likely to affect you.

Types of Drugs Influencing Sleep

Greek mythology holds that the god of sleep, Hypnos, flew around dispensing poppy stalks to eagerly awaiting gods and mortals. Dr. Ernest Hartmann believes, "The juice of the poppy was perhaps the first 'sleeping pill,' and it is not an exaggeration to say that the poppy (especially its derivatives, morphine and heroin) has been and still is worshiped almost as a god." The descendants of Hypnos have thrived by generating a vast array of sleep-inducing chemicals, so that today there are over 200 commercially available brands in the United States alone.

There also is a plethora of medications that just as forcibly hasten sleep but that are not called "sleeping pills," because this is not their principal function. For example, though antihistamines are used mainly for allergies, many of them are potent soporifics. Add alcohol and illegal drugs like marijuana to this cornucopia, and you have an endless number of sleep-altering substances.

Although somewhat arbitrarily, you can divide this pharmacological morass into four groups: (a) *over-the-counter* (OTC) or non-prescription sleep aids; (b) prescription sleeping pills or *hypnotics,* whose chief purpose is to produce sleep; (c) prescription drugs that, in addition to their primary function, also facilitate sleep—this group of *secondary sleep inducers* includes sedatives, antidepressants, antihistamines, major tranquilizers, and narcotics; and (d) alcohol, marijuana, and other *recreational substances* that have also been used for sleep. A fifth group, *stimulants,* such as amphetamines and cocaine, deserve attention because of their popularity and their disruptive effects on sleep.

In this chapter we'll look at each of these groups, seeing what they do and how they work. We'll examine their advantages and hazards. I'll discuss how you can know when you're hooked on sleeping pills and how you can get off them. I'll also specify those occasional circumstances in which you might use sleeping pills with reasonable safety and effectiveness. But before I go into detail about any particular medication, it's important for you to understand that there's much more to a drug than the chemicals that compose it.

Genies-in-the-Bottle

For the first time Mrs. Grant visits Dr. Sebastian. She complains, "I can't sleep." After performing an examination, he reassuringly tells her that she is free of any other medical problems, and dashes off a prescription for sleeping pills. Beaming confidence, he says, "These will do the trick. If you have any difficulties, give me a call." She thanks Dr. Sebastian and says, "Good-bye."

This ostensibly straightforward and mundane exchange, masks an intricate psychological drama that is staged a hundred times every day throughout the nation. Even a superficial examination of this situation reveals many unanswered questions.

Why does Mrs. Grant see a doctor in the first place? Not everybody who has a sleepless night consults a physician. Mrs. Grant decides to spend the time, money, and effort to visit a doctor, not just because she has insomnia, but more important, because she is sufficiently upset by it and expects that a physician can help her.

What does Mrs. Grant mean when she complains, "I can't sleep"? Maybe she's just fatigued and wants relief. But if so, has her tiredness been occurring for a year, a month, a week, or a day? Why did she consult the doctor *today*? Why not earlier, or later? Did she begin to feel helpless about her lack of sleep? Did a friend suggest, "Hey, that sounds terrible, you better see a doctor"? Is she really worried that she has another illness, like diabetes or cancer, that is producing her insomnia? Is she too scared to say so, fearing that she'll receive bad news, and does she therefore sidestep the issue by making a relatively innoculous complaint like "I can't sleep"? Is she more comfortable presenting herself as somebody with insomnia rather than saying, "My life is a mess. I'm anxious, depressed, and fearful. I'm getting old, I can't remember things, my children have left me, my husband ignores me, my boss is about to fire me, I'm flunking night school, and I'm ugly. That's why I can't sleep!" Mrs. Grant does have insomnia. But when she says, "I can't sleep," she may be concerned with more than just sleeplessness.

What does Mrs. Grant expect from Dr. Sebastian? Does she simply want him to quickly give her a pill? If so, how? Does she want an honest presentation? "These pills can work for only a week, will aggravate your fatigue, and are potentially addicting." Or, would she prefer reassurance? "These pills are really going to help you sleep. They're safe, and you'll feel tip-top in no time flat!" If Mrs. Grant wants the less comforting but more honest approach, why does she not inquire about the dangers of taking these pills? Is she ignorant? Unlikely, for everybody knows that medications have side effects. But maybe she is afraid to ask, sensing or assuming that Dr. Sebastian will be displeased by being questioned. If so, no wonder she can't share her concerns with him. Maybe she doesn't want to hear that the pills are hazardous. Does she want Dr. Sebastian to be a fatherly Marcus Welby, a whimsical Hawkeye Pierce, or an authoritative Ben Casey? Does she want Dr. Sebastian to ignore or to explore what really troubles her? Having a leave-well-enough-alone attitude, maybe she's relieved that Dr. Sebastian did not muck around in her mind or refer her to a "shrink"? On the other hand, maybe she yearns to have Dr. Sebastian talk with her but is too timid to say so?

How does Mrs. Grant view her taking of sleeping pills? Does she see the pills as merely a convenient and quick solution to an annoying problem? Or does she take them with the expectation that life's problems will disappear? "If I can sleep with these pills, I will no longer feel tired, old, anxious, and depressed. My children and husband will love me, I'll do better at work, and I'll even look more attractive." Perhaps the sleeping pill represents a capitulation, a final defeat? "I hate pills, but I'm so desperate, I must resort to them even though I know they're dangerous."

Why does Dr. Sebastian ignore all of these questions by simply dispensing the pills? Maybe he's obtuse or doesn't know any better. Maybe he doesn't care. But why not? Maybe he's rushed, having a dozen anxious patients with more serious complaints crowding his waiting room. Maybe the problem of insomnia does not capture his interest nearly as much as do the illnesses of those twelve patients eagerly awaiting him. Maybe he intuitively assesses that Mrs. Grant doesn't want to talk about her troubles or hear the truth about sleeping pills. Maybe Mrs. Grant unconsciously reminds Dr. Sebastian of his wife or mother, with whom he has just had an argument. Maybe he's not in the mood to hear another "Mrs. Sebastian" complain to him. Maybe he dismisses Mrs. Grant as "just another hypochrondriacal female." Maybe he wishes to hide his own sense of impotence in treating nagging sleep problems. Doctors want to believe they can cure. But when they can't, to avoid feeling helpless, they often feel compelled to *do* something. To many physicians, giving a pill is "doing," talking is not. Dr. Sebastian may be rationalizing: "I really can't help her, and I don't want to waste her time and mine; so I'll just give her the pills she wants."

What started as a simple complaint of "I can't sleep," followed by a routine prescription for hypnotics, is really a complicated unspoken psychological conspiracy between Mrs. Grant and Dr. Sebastian. Both have covertly agreed not to address a host of emotional issues whose importance clearly overshadows the technical questions regarding the type and dose of the sleeping pills themselves.

Nevertheless, the centerpiece of this psychodrama is the sleeping pill. It serves both of them as a convenient shortcut for avoiding the expression of their fears and expectations. Sleeping pills act as genies-in-a-bottle because they spare the two protagonists from discussing a myriad of sensitive topics.

The other genies-in-the-bottle are named *placebo effects*. A placebo (Latin for "I will please") is a biologically inactive substance, which masquerades as a real medication. Placebo effects refer to a person's responses to this fake drug, taken in the belief that it is the genuine item. How a person reacts to a placebo is determined solely by his *expectations* of how the authentic drug would affect him.

If a patient thinks he's received a tranquilizer, when he's really taken a placebo, he may experience nothing except disappointment and surprise that the medication was ineffective. But there is a good chance that he will genuinely feel calm. This *positive placebo response* occurs because he naturally *expects* to be relaxed by a real tranquilizer. He also may have a *negative placebo response* by developing "side effects"—dry mouth, dizziness, or anything else he *expects* that drug to produce.

These positive and negative placebo responses are really felt; they are not "just in his head." Although only reacting to a placebo, the subject may feel as calm or as dizzy as he would in response to an authentic tranquilizer. The more suggestible the person, the more powerful his placebo reactions. But it would be misleading to believe that only very suggestible individuals experience placebo responses. Because everyone expects something to happen when taking a drug, many perfectly rational people develop placebo reactions. Therefore, unless it is studied scientifically, it is unclear if your response to a medication derives from the drug's placebo effects, its biological actions, or both. When touted as a sleeping pill, a mere placebo can become a potent sleep inducer.

Not only do placebos exert powerful effects along the lines anticipated by the patient, but also in ways he would have little ability to control or even know about. For example, Dr. Ernest Hartmann found that healthy male volunteers had decreased REM sleep when first given a sham hypnotic. They even displayed a greater proportion of REM sleep a few days after the placebo was discontinued— the precise time when REM rebound (see Chapter 2, p. 51–52) occurs after stopping many genuine hypnotics. Evidently, your psychological expectations of a sleeping pill can alter your physiological responses to a placebo, even if you're unaware of them.

Consequently, *anything* called a "sleeping pill" can induce sleep, because regardless of its actual contents, it encapsulates our expectations. Placebo responses are important to consider when evaluating the usefulness of any medication, especially over-the-counter drugs.

Over-the-Counter Sleep Aids

In 1978, ten million Americans paid $27 million for one of over a hundred brands of over-the-counter (OTC) sleep aids. According to the 1970–71 National Survey on Drug Acquisition and Use, 6 percent of the adult population bought OTC sleeping pills, while 3.5 percent purchased hypnotics. These groups did not overlap; those who used OTC sleep aids did not take hypnotics, and users of hypnotics did not consume OTC sleep aids.

Aggressive advertising partially accounts for the popularity of OTC sleeping pills. Every night, television assaults us with yawning middle-aged housewives relieved that their Sominex, Nytol, or whatever will grace them with blissful slumber. In 1978, $5 million and $2.5 million were spent foisting Sominex and Nytol respectively on the public.

A purpose of this commercial onslaught is to acquaint you with the *name* of a product, rather than with the drug itself. The reason is simple: Although the brand name remains the same, the actual contents of the drug frequently change. For example, the Food and Drug Administration (FDA) recalled OTC sleep aids containing methapyrilene (the antihistamine formerly in Sominex, Nytol, Excedrin P.M., Compoz, Sleep-Eze, and many others) because the National Cancer Institute concluded that it caused liver cancer in rats and mice, and presumably in people. Subsequently, methapyrilene was replaced by a related compound, pyrilamine, a supposedly milder, safer, but less soporific antihistamine. Similarly, when the FDA decided that the scopolamine in sleep aids was potentially dangerous and probably ineffective, it was quietly removed from most OTC sleep aids. When an advertisement claims that an OTC agent is "new and improved," it may not necessarily mean that the drug is more beneficial, but merely that it's less hazardous.

Consequently, if you are going to purchase an OTC sleeping pill, the brand name will not tell you what you're actually buying. Instead, you have to note the chemical names of the substances written in small print on the package in order to know what you're taking. It's quite possible that your drugstore still carries the old Sominex instead of its newly formulated version. That's why it's important to read labels. If you're unable to make head nor tail of, let alone pronounce, those chemical names, ask your pharmacist for advice.

Before you spend your money on these products, remember that so far the FDA has not determined that *any* OTC sleep aids are worthwhile. At vest, the FDA has ruled that currently (1980) there is insufficient evidence to indicate whether these drugs meet reasonable standards of safety and efficacy. Although most, but certainly not all, investigations have shown that OTC sleep aids are ineffective, further research will be required before the FDA can approve these products or remove them from the marketplace.

In the meantime, such information as does exist suggests that if OTC sleep aids are helpful, it is largely due to their placebo effects. Drs. David Davis and Ernest Hartmann conducted experiments with two groups of subjects comparing the usefulness of no medication, a placebo, and Sominex (with methapyrilene). The first group of subjects were men, aged twenty-one to forty-five. The second group were forty-five- to sixty-five-year-old women, who as a class are the greatest consumers of OTC sleep aids. (No wonder commercials for OTC sleep aids are targeted at them.) It turned out that only the women fell asleep significantly more quickly on Sominex. But the study also revealed that whereas the men took longer to drop off on placebo than on no medication, the women did just the reverse. The most likely explanation for these peculiar findings is that for the women the pharmacological efficacy of Sominex was enhanced considerably because of their favorable expectations of the drug. On the other hand, being leery about the medication to begin with, the men were less apt to doze off sooner with the drug. Consequently, since OTC sleep aids are innocuous or only mildly beneficial, your *expectations* of them, whether positive or negative, will be a major factor in determining how effective they will be for you.

Although placebo responses do play a significant role, OTC "sleepers" are not placebos. For inexplicable reasons, some of them consist of thiamine (vitamin B_1) and passionflower extract. More often, however, the OTC sleep aids sitting on your pharmacist's shelves contain one or a combination of four types of substances, each having various degrees of usefulness and safety.

BROMIDES   In order to be effective, doses larger than those found in OTCs (e.g., Alva-Tranquil) would be needed. Furthermore, several nights of continuous use must elapse before you can achieve the blood levels necessary to induce sleep. But if bromides are taken for an extended period, or if too many pills are consumed at once, severe mental disturbances are likely to occur, especially in the elderly. Devoid of any redeeming qualities, and also potentially dangerous, bromides have recently been removed by most manufacturers from their products. But since leftover bromide OTC sleep aids are still available, the old bromide "Let the buyer beware!" remains applicable.

SCOPOLAMINE Why this drug was ever put into sleep aids escapes me. Whereas they contain too little of the drug to be effective, they do possess enough scopolamine to cause dryness of the mouth and mucous membranes, blurred vision, constipation, irregular heart beats, and stomach distress. Those who are particularly sensitive to the drug, especially the elderly, can develop severe memory impairment, confusion, and disorientation. Scopolamine is particularly dangerous for those with glaucoma, prostate difficulties, and heart disease. Some patients in severe pain who take scopolamine sleep aids are apt to become restless and delirious. So too are patients who simultaneously use antidepressants, major tranquilizers, or any drugs that cause dry mouth, such as cold tablets. At doses higher than those in sleep aids, scopolamine reduces REM sleep; once stopped, it produces REM rebound with nightmares and insomnia.

Pharmaceutical houses have generally complied with the FDA's attempts to eliminate scopolamine-containing OTC sleeping remedies from the market. But old bottles of these drugs remain in many stores; as with bromides, make sure you don't buy them by mistake.

PAIN RELIEVERS (*analgesics*) Aspirin, salicylamide (a weaker version of aspirin), or acetaminophen are often placed in OTC sleep aids. The flimsy justification for incorporating these drugs is that pain may cause insomnia. True, but so what? If pain is disturbing your sleep, then treat the pain! The FDA concurs. (The old nostrum of taking aspirin for sleep is equally nonsensical. Aspirin is great for many conditions, but not for insomnia.)

ANTIHISTAMINES This group, which was once chiefly represented by methapyrilene, now includes pyrilamine, phenytoloxamine, diphenhydramine, and doxylamine. In larger (prescription) doses, antihistamines temporarily induce sleep and diminish REM. But the small quantities of antihistamines in OTC sleep aids render them minimally, if at all, effective. Although the subject has been insufficiently researched, the investigations that have been conducted suggest that antihistamine sleep aids may be useful for mild but not for severe insomnia.

Antihistamines principally alleviate allergies; grogginess is a mere side effect. Therefore, a side effect is actually being used to foster sleep. This wouldn't be too hard to swallow, but the drowsiness can persist into daytime, making driving and working with machinery hazardous. What's more, grogginess is often magnified two to four times when used concurrently with alcohol. If you have asthma, glaucoma, or an enlarged prostate, you should take antihistamines only under a doctor's close supervision.

Given all their hazards, and whatever nominal sleep-inducing qualities they possess, I cannot see any good reason for employing most OTC sleep aids. But if you wish to try them, remember the following points:

• *They are all dangerous to children*. Besides warning about the risk of accidental overdosing, the manufacturers specifically state: "Do not give to children under twelve years of age."

• *Check with your physician if you have any illnesses or are using any other prescription or even nonprescription medications*. The ingredients of OTC sleep aids may aggravate your disease or adversely interact with other drugs. For example, because many cold tablets also contain antihistamines, they, in combination with an OTC sleep aid, may give you more sleep than you bargained for.

• *Carefully follow the instructions on the package*. Doubling the dose may produce toxicity without enhancing efficacy.

• *These drugs should be consumed only for occasional difficulties in falling asleep*. They will not alleviate middle insomnia. Taking these drugs continuously for more than two weeks may aggravate sleeplessness or mask and complicate an underlying illness.

• *Buy OTCs that contain only an antihistamine*. Although I would prefer that you not use any OTC sleep aids, those with antihistamines alone have the best chance for success, especially for those persons with mild insomnia.

• *Compare costs*. Prices for pharmacologically identical substances can vary enormously. When checking this out, however, make sure you compare the same dose of the same ingredient. Many OTC sleep aids suggest taking two tablets, others only one.

• *Learn more*. Available at most major libraries and at all medical school libraries is the *Handbook of Nonprescription Drugs* (Washington, D.C.: American Pharmaceutical Association, 1979). It's the best source of information about OTC sleep aids. Since the chemicals in these drugs are perpetually being changed, make sure you consult the latest edition, which in 1979 was the sixth.

Madison Avenue ingenuity will undoubtedly continue to promote wonderful "new formula" over-the-counter sleep aids. The more skeptical you are about these products, the safer you and your family will be. If you "need" to take something before going to bed, the tryptophan in a cup of warm milk (Chapter 4) is more effective, and certainly safer and cheaper than any OTC sleep remedy.

Hypnotics: Their Effects on Sleep

Hypnotics do not act specifically on the body's "sleep center." Instead, they exert a *general* depressant effect throughout the brain. Besides diminishing alertness and inducing sleep, one sleeping pill dulls the senses and slows respiration. In large doses hypnotics cause anesthesia, coma, and death. Therefore, sleep facilitation is a mere by-product of a hypnotic's overall depressant influence on the brain.

Initially, all hypnotics put you to sleep within ten to thirty minutes. With the exception of Dalmane, however, a hypnotic's soporific power wears off after five to seven nights. In other words, after they have been used for several consecutive days, most sleeping pills are pharmacologically worthless. If, after a week, a hypnotic other than Dalmane still *appears* to promote sleep, it is principally because of its placebo effect and, as mentioned in Chapter 4, its value as a bedtime ritual. Dalmane is the only hypnotic that genuinely facilitates sleep for up to a month. Whether Dalmane is useful beyond thirty days is unknown. Therefore, if you have difficulties in falling asleep, hypnotics might be useful, but for only a brief period.

Whereas initially all hypnotics can put you to sleep, only some of them can remedy middle-of-the-night awakenings (i.e., middle insomnia). For example, chloral hydrate and Doriden cannot alleviate middle insomnia. On the other hand, Dalmane, the barbiturate hypnotics, and possibly Noludar and Quaalude can minimize nocturnal awakenings. Except for Dalmane, even those "sleepers" that initially reduce middle-of-the-night awakenings will fizzle out within a week. Furthermore, the continued use of all hypnotics is more likely to cause then to prevent middle insomnia.

To varying extents, almost every hypnotic alters sleep stages. As I detailed in Chapter 2, barbiturates first suppress REM sleep. But within several days the body "makes up for" this loss and an excess of REM gushes forth—the so-called "REM rebound" effect. From the outset of this chapter you may recall that shortly after Howard began using Nembutal, his sleep was disrupted by repeated nightmares of Toby lying disfigured in a frozen cubicle. Although he didn't know it, Howard was experiencing REM rebound. Except for Dalmane and chloral hydrate, *all* hypnotics produce REM rebound after a few nights.

The adverse effects of hypnotics can be mild and transitory or severe and prolonged, depending on how much and for how long they are used. If you take one capsule, you may experience minimal discomfort for a day or two. You might feel groggy the next morning, have more trouble dropping off the next evening, or sleep restlessly that night. With habitual use, all of these symptoms will be intensified, and middle insomnia will eventually add to your sleeplessness. Chronic hypnotic abusers like Howard quickly discover that the most expeditious way to dampen the effects of REM rebound is to increase the dose. This short-term "solution," however, merely delays and compounds the problem. The perpetual pill popper now confronts a dilemma: He either endures many nights when it's nearly impossible to sleep or he capitulates by taking more medication. The best way to avoid this dilemma is not to get into it.

Unlike every other hypnotic, chloral hydrate causes little if any disruption of normal sleep stages. But unless the dose is raised, after a week of continued use, chloral hydrate loses its sleep-inducing capacities. The problem with escalating the dose is that by doing so you can easily put yourself to sleep—forever. Chloral hydrate's usual therapeutic dose is one to one and a half grams. As little as four grams can be lethal.

Although Dalmane, the most popular of the hypnotics, has a nominal effect on REM, it substantially reduces stage 4 sleep. This loss of deep sleep, coupled with Dalmane's (and most other hypnotics') tendency to linger in the bloodstream, often results in a hazy, numbed, hungover feeling the next day. Paradoxically, Dalmane may produce the very fatigue you hoped it would eliminate. Feeling "drugged," you're tempted to nap during the day, which in turn makes it harder to fall asleep at night.

The *continued* use of any hypnotic aggravates rather than alleviates insomnia. Whether by causing REM rebound, by decreasing stage 4 sleep, by remaining too long in the bloodstream, or by quickly losing their effectiveness, all sleeping pills eventually disturb sleep and dull wakefulness. The hypnotic-taking insomniac is likely to blame his inadequate sleep rather than the drug for his daytime fatigue. After all, it is perfectly reasonable to assume that sleeping pills help you sleep. (It might be more accurate to call hypnotics "sleepless pills" than "sleeping pills.") You might naturally, but incorrectly, believe that another tablet will put you to sleep. Indeed, for a couple of days the additional medication will enable you to sleep. But when your sleep becomes chaotic again and you feel desperate, you're apt to remember this immediate benefit and overlook that the hypnotic is the real culprit. Being frustrated during a restless night, you're likely to be overwhelmed by the urge to do something—anything—to knock yourself out. "Do something" usually translates into "Take another pill." Instead of giving in to this understandable but impulsive and short-sighted response, if you feel compelled to "do something," implement the suggestions in the preceding five chapters. These nondrug alternatives may or may not bring instant relief. But with time, and unlike hypnotics that eventually cause insomnia, natural methods will effectively, repeatedly, and safely allow you to sleep.

Hypnotics: Their Hazards

Using any medication places you in jeopardy. Even the lowly aspirin can cause you to bleed to death. But the fact remains that people gobble aspirin all the time; their headaches vanish and they don't die. In deciding to take *any* drug, you must weigh its potential benefits and risks. When evaluating its risks, you have to know not only what potential hazards exist, but also the likelihood of their occurring, given your particular circumstances. The chance of your bleeding from two aspirin is infinitesimal, unless you have a severe ulcer, in which case the risk might be substantial. Drugs, then, are neither safe nor dangerous; they are only relatively safe or relatively dangerous.

Later in this chapter, Table 9.1 details the major side effects caused by the most widely used hypnotic agents. Some of these problems are so common or so crucial, however, that they deserve further elaboration.

PREGNANCY Sleeping pills *must* not be taken during pregnancy. Hypnotics readily pass through the placenta and freely circulate into the fetal system. The fetus is defenseless against the onslaught of the drug. What is one pill to you is like twenty to fifty pills to the fetus. Its metabolic system is poorly equipped to handle the drug's depressant effects on the brain.

Although there is no firm proof that sleeping pills cause congenital abnormalities, there is some evidence that exposure to benzodiazepine (e.g., Dalmane, Valium, Librium) gives rise to birth defects, especially cleft lip. Barbiturates taken during pregnancy are associated with an increased risk of improperly formed cardiovascular systems at birth and brain tumors later in childhood. These problems are most likely to occur if the mother uses sleeping pills during the first three months of pregnancy.

Pregnant mothers who habitually consume hypnotics may give birth to addicted children. These newborns begin life by undergoing potentially lethal withdrawal symptoms. Watching such children is among the most chilling and pathetic experiences I've ever had.

BREAST FEEDING Sleeping pills and daytime sedatives (especially Valium) are carried in breast milk. Although you might need a sedative while you're nursing, your child doesn't; use the relaxation exercises in Chapter 5 instead.

GROGGINESS The soporific effects of most sleeping pills do not completely wear off by the time you awake. How long daytime fatigue due to hypnotics persists depends on how quickly the drug is metabolized and eliminated from your body. One of the few advantages of Nodular and Placidyl is that most of their ingredients are out of your system by morning. By contrast, half of the active chemicals in barbiturate hypnotics linger for fourteen to ninety-six hours after you take them. The major active metabolite (by-product) of Dalmane remains in the body for two to four days. Therefore, if you take hypnotics on consecutive nights, new drugs are being added to your system before the old drugs can be eliminated. As a result, with continued sleeping-pill use, hypnotics accumulate, thereby compounding daytime fatigue. Even a single dose of most sleeping pills can impair alertness and performance for eighteen hours.

If you're a habitual user, you become acclimated, after a while, to walking around in a fog. Your thinking is not sharp, your reflexes are not swift, and your movements are not precise. You might become so accustomed to this hypnotic-induced haze that eventually you're unaware of being in it; you fail to recognize that you're no longer operating at peak efficiency. Even after taking one pill, you may not appreciate on the next day the subtle impairment in your thinking and functioning. Therefore, *if you've used a sleeping pill in the past twenty-four hours, you must be extra cautious about driving, operating machinery, crossing streets, and the like.*

DRUG DEPENDENCY   So as not to offend the purchasing public, television offensively transmits a one-sided view of addiction. By only portraying addicts as slimy heroin-shooting psychopaths, television "forgets" to present the typical sleeping-pill addict—a pressured executive, a bored house-wife, a "workaholic" physician, an elderly farmer, a high-school cheerleader. Like Howard, these decent and productive citizens have little in common with half-crazed needle freaks. But unlike heroin junkies, *sleeping-pill addicts can die from withdrawal symptoms.* Hypnotic abusers may not even know they're addicted.

Drug dependency can be psychological and physical. And although there are no universally recognized definitions of these types of drug dependency, the following descriptions are widely accepted. *Psychological dependency* occurs when a person relies on a mind-altering substance to cope more effectively with his life. When the dose of the drug needs to be increased in order to obtain the same psychological or physical effects, *tolerance* has set in. In other words, the same amount of the drug no longer yields as good a "high" or as satisfying a sleep. *Withdrawal* is a stereotypical pro-gression of symptoms that occurs when the consumption of a substance is substantially decreased or stopped. When tolerance has developed and suddenly discontinuing the drug would bring on withdrawal, *physical dependency* exists. In this context the terms "addiction" and "physical dependency" are used interchangeably.

Howard's experiences illustrate these concepts. When he felt incapable of sleep without Nembutal, he was already psychologically dependent. By the time the drug's soporific effects had worn off, tolerance had developed. Now he required an extra capsule to fall asleep. When he became tolerant to two capsules, larger doses, boosted by the whiskey, were needed simply to doze off. Like a man hanging from a cliff, Howard knew that continued Nembutal use was necessary if he was to avoid plunging into the abyss. But after the fire, he fell. Because he and his doctors were focusing intensely on his near fatal burns, sleeping-pill abuse was the last thing on their minds. Routine blood tests do not even reveal drug use. Everybody, Howard included, assumed that his growing confusion, irritability, and restlessness were caused by his burns; it never occurred to them that these symptoms were a part of drug withdrawal. If it had, these symptoms as well as his epilepticlike seizures could have been prevented. Knowing that Howard was physically dependent on Nembutal, the physicians could have enabled him to withdraw comfortably and safely by giving him a gradually lowered dose of Nembutal.

All hypnotics produce psychological and physical dependency. Because all sleeping pills similarly depress the brain, people who withdraw from any hypnotic will undergo a similar ordeal. The list below shows the usual *sequence* of a full-blown withdrawal syndrome.

How Withdrawal Symptoms Typically Progress

Weakness	Light-headedness or dizziness
Restlessness	on standing up (due to a
Tremulousness	drop in blood pressure)
Insomnia	Rapid pulse and heart rates
Spasms of the eyelids	Anxiety
(blepharospasm)	Fever

Convulsions

Psychosis (may include visual hallucinations, confusion, paranoid thoughts, sensation of creeping ants on the skin,

auditory hallucinations, delirium)

Continued seizures (status epilepticus)

Death

The consistency and the quantity of hypnotic use largely determine how many of these symptoms will develop. Although taking an occasional pill may interfere with sleep the following night, genuine withdrawal does not ensue. If a single tablet is consumed almost every night for one or two weeks, even though tolerance may have set in and sleep will be disrupted for several evenings, no catastrophe will ensue. When a larger habit has been established, however, such as a month-long diet of 400 milligrams (or four capsules) of Nembutal a night, abruptly stopping or substantially reducing the amount of the drug results in weakness, tremulousness, insomnia, spasms of the eyelids, and severe dizziness. At 500 milligrams, 10 to 15 percent of the patients also become feverish, hallucinate, and convulse. With nightly habits greater than 900 milligrams, a majority of the patients become psychotic and 80 percent have seizures. Once convulsions begin, which can be anytime from sixteen hours to ten days after discontinuing the hypnotic, death itself may result.

Withdrawal symptoms can emerge at even lower doses, if the use of sleeping pills is accompanied by the steady consumption of alcohol, sedatives, or other hypnotics. Since all of these chemicals exert a similar effect on the nervous system, they intensify, when taken in concert, the severity of dependency and withdrawal. Because Howard was regularly imbibing a couple of nightcaps to wash down his sleeping pills, his "mere" 400-milligram habit produced withdrawal symptoms "worthy" of an 800-milligram or a 900-milligram habit.

I'm presenting this grizzly picture of hypnotic dependence to frighten you. I haven't exaggerated the danger of drug withdrawal; I've merely outlined the facts, and the facts *are* frightening. If you periodically take a sleeping pill, I don't want you to panic, just to be cautious.

When you've reached a point at which one pill (or actually one standard dose) no longer puts you to sleep, you've already developed tolerance. If you're still consuming only one pill, stop now, and, for heaven's sake, don't take any more. If you're now using two pills every night, taper yourself off the medication by taking one pill fewer every two weeks. If you're regularly using more than twice the normal dose, *do not stop the drug on your own;* you could precipitate withdrawal. Instead, consult your physician. If you don't have a doctor, get one. He can establish a schedule by which you come off the drug slowly, comfortably, and safely.

TOXICITY   Late at night in the emergency room of the Yale-New Haven Hospital, I watched Angie drift in and out of a coma. She was twenty years old. Her strong and attractive features seemed inappropriate to someone lying so helplessly on a stretcher. On regaining consciousness, she said that her boyfriend, who was reliably unreliable, had promised to take her camping for the weekend. But at the last minute, he canceled the venture and took off with a buddy to see a Yankee baseball game. Then Angie coldly counted and swallowed ten Doriden tablets. (For the past year she had regularly used them for sleep.) As she glanced at the intravenous fluids flowing into her arm, Angie lamented, "I only wanted to scare him. I never *really* intended to harm myself." She gently closed her eyes and returned to sleep. Twenty minutes later she died.

Angie's senseless death illustrates that whether a fatality results from an overdose depends on many factors, only one of them being the number of pill consumed.

Hypnotics vary enormously in their capacity to produce toxicity. If Angie had taken ten Dalmane instead of ten Doriden, she would still be alive. Toxicity will *not* develop from taking *any* hypnotic at double or even triple the normal therapeutic dose, unless other drugs are also being taken. In

larger amounts, however, sleeping pill toxicity is particularly common with chloral hydrate, Doriden, Quaalude, and
any of the barbiturate-type hypnotics. In terms of toxicity
only, Dalmane is the safest of all prescription sleeping pills.
Because all hypnotics depress the nervous system and therefore potentially interfere with breathing, persons with
respiratory ailments are particularly susceptible to the toxic
effects of sleeping pills. Being unable to metabolize and
eliminate chemicals from their bodies, people with liver and
kidney diseases are also at high risk. Numerous medications
adversely interact with hypnotics, especially oral anticoagu-
lants (blood thinners such as Coumadin), antidepressants
(e.g., Tofranil, Elavil), and anticholinergics (e.g., Donnatal,
Belladenal).

The elderly are in general so sensitive to hypnotics that
half the normal dose is usually sufficient to induce sleep.
(The elderly are also inclined to develop ''paradoxical
reactions''; that is, after taking a hypnotic, they become
restless and excited rather than tired.) Because older people
are likely to have at least one chronic disease and to be
taking medications, their chances of becoming toxic on
sleeping pills are greatly enhanced. In 1979 the National
Academy of Sciences recommended that physicians be especially cautious in prescribing hypnotics for the elderly.

When alcohol or sedatives are taken in conjunction with
hypnotics, the toxic effects of all of these chemicals are
magnified exponentially. In other words, mixing drugs, each
of which depresses the nervous system, creates a situation in
which $1 + 1 = 4$. On top of a sleeping pill, one drink feels
like three or four drinks. If taken separately, several shots of
whiskey (or a couple of sedatives) and two or three sleeping
pills would not produce any dire consequences. But if they
are taken together, serious toxicity and death can result.

The risk of an accidental fatality also increases with
continued drug use. Because tolerance develops more to the
soporific than to the lethal effects of sleeping pills, you can
readily underestimate the danger of taking additional tablets.
We know about all too many rock-music stars and other
show-business celebrities who falsely assumed that because

they no longer became sleepy or "high" on a few pills, they could take more of them with impunity.

Although you might exercise proper caution in using sleeping pills, children will not. Kids are apt to gobble down any drug in sight, possibly thinking they are delicious and chewy vitamins. Even if you personally don't have any small children, your visitors might. All medication, but especially sleeping pills, should therefore be kept in a safe place. So called "child-proof" bottles afford little protection. Only adults and pathologically clumsy children have difficulty opening them.

The hazards of sleeping pills are due as much to the person using them as to the drugs themselves. Pregnant and breast-feeding mothers simply have no business taking hypnotics. The elderly must be especially cautious. Accidents stemming from grogginess are usually caused by insufficient awareness that one is still slowed down by last night's medication. Physical dependency and toxicity result from poor judgment, from too little self-control, and from self-deception. If hypnotics are used properly, except for idiosyncratic allergies, daytime grogginess will be the most serious consequence. But since most sleeping pills lose their potency within five to seven days, they can be used only occasionally for overcoming insomnia. There's no question that nonpharmacological means of coping with sleeplessness are still the safest and most enduringly effective ones.

Hypnotics: Their Use

Why would anybody take (let alone pay for) a substance whose continued use leads to grogginess, insomnia, addiction, and toxicity? Conservatively, 5.7 percent of adult Americans are annually doing exactly that. But why? It could be that these nine million people are unaware of the hazards. Undoubtedly, lack of information is part of the answer. But in my experience, most people are like Howard; although they may be ignorant of the specifics, they know that using hypnotics involves risks. So why do these potentially dangerous medications still hold such great appeal? The reasons are numerous and complex. Two of these motivations, however, seem to lie at the heart of the matter.

Use of hypnotics is *convenient*. We seek instant replays, instant food, instant pleasures, instant solutions, instant cures. We also wish to expend as little effort as possible in obtaining these goodies. We learn about complicated foreign or domestic issues by passively watching a sixty-second televised synopsis rather than by listening to an in-depth discussion or reading the newspaper. We treat our health as we do our politics. We want instant results that demand little or no energy. Natural methods for alleviating insomnia take time. Sleeping pills work immediately. Natural methods require effort, sleeping pills do not.

Hypnotics *work,* or, more accurately, they are believed to work. Natural methods simply do not enjoy the scientific mystique associated with hypnotics. Because drugs are the product of an awesome technology, people have faith in their capacity to relieve symptoms. We not only believe that hypnotics are powerful, they *are* powerful. Experience teaches that with hypnotics there is no shilly-shalling around; you take one, and it puts you to sleep. Over and over again, I'm struck by how patients will politely listen to instructions for overcoming insomnia naturally, only to ask, "But what about the *real* stuff?" The "real stuff," of course, is medication.

Therefore, despite all the hazards and limitations inherent in the use of hypnotics, sleeping pills retain their popularity because they *are* a convenient and powerful way to fall asleep. People know this, because it's true; there's no point in pretending otherwise.

In deciding whether to use sleeping pills, you must first weigh the risks involved, appreciate that they can be only temporarily helpful, and recognize that natural methods are the only permanent remedies for insomnia.

Employing hypnotics is, in my opinion, justified under only two circumstances. First, hypnotics can be helpful for coping with an *occasional* (i.e., no more than once a week) sleepless night. Even then, make sure you won't generate more problems than you're trying to solve. If you're anxious and unable to sleep because you have an exam tomorrow, I would *not* recommend your using a sleeping pill. Although the drug would put you to sleep, you'd be apt to feel tired and to have more difficulties concentrating the next day. Even though Noludar and Placidyl leave your system faster than other hypnotics, and therefore produce less daytime grogginess, there is no way of predicting how you specifically will respond to the drug. Consequently, it's inadvisable for you to use hypnotics the night before any day on which you need to be especially clear-headed, whether it's for taking a big exam, interviewing for an important job, or driving long distances. On the other hand, if you are unable to fall asleep and will be lounging around your home tomorrow, a hypnotic could be taken with relative safety. Because it rarely produces a hangover, has a minimal effect on sleep stages, and is relatively inexpensive, chloral hydrate is particularly helpful for such episodic use.

Second, during periods of considerable emotional upheaval, Dalmane can be taken on consecutive evenings, but for no more than a week. Continuing sleeping-pill use beyond this time is courting psychological dependence, which, in turn, can lead to physical dependence. Dalmane is preferable for continued use principally because it maintains its effectiveness longer than any other hypnotic. But once again, you must be extra cautious about daytime grogginess, because Dalmane accumulates in your body when taken repeatedly. If the emotional crisis and its accompanying insomnia persist for more than a week, medication should be stopped and nonpharmacological remedies instituted.

Although I prefer chloral hydrate for episodic use and Dalmane for short-term use, it is possible that your physician will prescribe other medications. He may have a good reason for doing so: You may, for example, be allergic to chloral hydrate or Dalmane, or you may have an illness or take medications that preclude your using them. No one drug is best for everybody under every circumstance. On the other hand, your doctor may be relatively unfamiliar with sleeping pills. Although you can evaluate your physician's bedside manner, you are less equipped to assess his pharmacological sophistication. Nevertheless, by possessing as much information as possible about the most widely prescribed hypnotics, you'll be in a better position to know if your doctor is giving you the proper medication. To make such a determination, you should judge the hypnotic by the following five criteria:

1. The hypnotic should have few side effects.
2. It should become toxic only at very high doses.
3. It should have a minimal effect on sleep stages.
4. The hypnotic should reduce middle-of-the-night awakenings as well as put you to sleep effectively.
5. It should have a brief "half-life"—which refers to the time it takes for half of the drug to leave your system. A hypnotic with a short half-life will produce less daytime grogginess.

According to these guidelines there is no ideal sleeping pill. You and your physician must select between less than fully desirable alternatives.

Table 9.1 lists the most widely prescribed hypnotics, their generic names, chemical classes, therapeutic doses, actions (including effects on sleep stages, half-lives, duration of effectiveness, influences on nocturnal awakenings), side effects, and precautions. Before using any sleeping pill, however, carefully review this table as well as the following Dos and Don'ts":

• *Do* ask your physician about the drug's side effects. If he tells you there aren't any, mention the hazards cited here.

• *Do* ask your doctor if the hypnotic will interfere with other medication you might be taking or aggravate any illness you might have.

• *Do* ask your doctor to prescribe a generic substitute for the more expensive brand-name hypnotic. Because of patent requirements, however, generic equivalents exist only for some sleeping pills. When generic substitutes are available, purchasing them can save you as much as 50 percent.

- *Do* insure that your pharmacist gives you the less costly generic drug. Because of limited space and the desire to avoid extra paper work, he might carry only the brand-name product. Any pharmacist can order a generic substitute that he does not have in stock.

- *Do* shop around and compare prices, whether you're using a generic or a brand-name hypnotic. In my neighborhood one hundred 15-milligram Dalmane cost from eleven to twenty dollars (in 1980).

- *Do* take the sleeping pill about twenty minutes before retiring.

- *Do* make sure to use a sleeping pill that reduces nocturnal awakenings if you have middle insomnia that is not due to any condition mentioned in Chapter 8.

- *Do* learn about the hypnotic you're taking. Consult *the* standard text on medications, Goodman and Gilman's *The Pharmacological Basis of Therapeutics,* fifth edition (New York: Macmillan, 1975), in your public or medical-school libraries. Another excellent, and certainly more readable, source is Dr. Ernest Hartmann's *The Sleeping Pill* (New Haven: Yale, 1978).

- *Don't* use anybody else's sleeping pills. Take only hypnotics prescribed for *you* by *your* doctor.

- *Don't* be timid about requesting information from your doctor. If he brushes aside your questions or resents answering them, you need another physician more than a sleeping pill.

- *Don't* refill a prescription without your doctor's explicit approval.

- *Don't* take the full therapeutic dose mentioned in Table 9.1 if you're over sixty years old. Instead, use half the dose, unless your physician says otherwise.

- *Don't* take sleeping pills on the same night that your spouse takes a sleeping pill.

- *Don't* drink, take sedatives, or narcotics when using hypnotics.

- *Don't* take hypnotics in the middle of the night.

- *Don't* use a drug to sleep during a plane trip.

9.1/COMMONLY USED HYPNOTICS

BRAND NAME(S)	GENERIC NAME (CHEMICAL CLASS)	USUAL THERAPEUTIC DOSE	ACTIONS
AMYTAL	Amobarbital (barbiturate)	100–200 mgs.*	Decreased REM with REM rebound; hypnotic action lasts 8–11 hours; half-life is 14–42 hours; wears off in 5–7 nights; reduces nocturnal awakenings

Comment: Although it is one of the better barbiturates, all barbiturates should be avoided.

| BUTISOL | Butabarbital (barbiturate) | 50–100 mgs. | Decreased REM with REM rebound; hypnotic action lasts 5–6 hours; half-life is unknown; wears off in 5–7 nights; reduces nocturnal awakenings |

Comment: There are better hypnotics than barbiturates.

SIDE EFFECTS	PRECAUTIONS
Hangover; lethargy; allergic reactions, such as skin blotches, swelling and itchiness, especially in patients with asthma, urticaria, or angioneurotic edema; confusion, marked agitation and excitement, especially in the elderly; dizziness; rashes; nausea; vomiting; diarrhea; headaches; fever; depression	Toxic dose is about 10 gms.* Should not be used by patients allergic to barbiturates. Must not be taken by patients with porphyria or during pregnancy, especially in the first three months; not to be taken by breast-feeding mothers; should be used in reduced doses for patients with liver, kidney, and respiratory diseases; may cause excitement in patients with uncontrollable pain; inhibits the effectiveness of oral anticoagulants, requiring these blood thinners to be monitored closely by your doctor; can lead to psychological and physical dependency; should not be taken with alcohol, narcotics, or sedatives; can decrease alertness, making driving and working with machines dangerous; should not be used by children under 15
Same as with Amytal	Same as with Amytal

Table continues on next page

9.1 / *continued*

BRAND NAME(S)	GENERIC NAME (CHEMICAL CLASS)	USUAL THERA-PEUTIC DOSE	ACTIONS
DALMANE	Flurazepam (benzodiazepine)	15–30 mgs. (preferably 15 mgs., especially in the elderly)	At 30 mgs. REM is unaffected; at 60 mgs. there is a slight decrease of REM, but without REM rebound; de-creased stage 4; hypnotic action lasts 7–8 hours; half-life of major active me-tabolite (by-product) is 47–100 hours; known to be ef-fective up to 30 days; reduces noc-turnal awakenings
DORIDEN	Glutethimide (piperidinedione)	500 mgs. (may be repeated, but not within 4 hours of awakening)	Barely induces sleep, and it even loses this ability in 5–7 nights; pain fur-ther decreases ef-fectiveness; de-creased REM with REM rebound; hyp-notic action lasts 4–8 hours; half-life is 10 hours; does not reduce nocturnal awakenings

Comment: Dalmane is the most efficacious of the hypnotics, especially for continued use.

Comment: Perhaps more than with any other hyp-notic, because Doriden's potential for inducing sleep is so low and that for producing toxicity and death is so high, I wish the FDA would remove it from the marketplace altogether!

SIDE EFFECTS	PRECAUTIONS
Hangover; lethargy; weakness; allergic reactions; dizziness; staggering; loss of muscle coordination and falling down, especially in the elderly and debilitated; headache; heartburn; nausea; vomiting; diarrhea; constipation; palpitations; chest, stomach, body, and joint pains; excitability and agitation, especially in the elderly. *Rare:* Decreased white blood cells (for fighting infections); sweating; flushes; blurred vision; burning eyes; faintness; shortness of breath; rashes; itching; dry mouth and throat; bitter taste; excessive salivation; loss of appetite; slurred speech; euphoria; depression; confusion; hallucinations	Toxic dose exceeds 3 gms.; can impair alertness for one or two days, making driving and machine work dangerous; not to be used if allergic to Dalmane; do not take with alcohol, narcotics, or sedatives; not to be used during pregnancy, especially in the first three months; not to be taken by breast-feeding mothers; should be used cautiously by those with liver or kidney diseases; may be habit forming; not recommended for children under 15
Hangover; lethargy; allergic skin rashes; dermititis. *Rare:* Nausea, excitement, and agitation, especially in the elderly; blurred vision; decreased platelets (for clotting) and red and white blood cells; abdominal distress; headache	Toxic dose can be 5 gms.; readily leads to psychological and physical dependency; not to be used if allergic to Doriden; not to be taken by pregnant or nursing mothers; very dangerous to use with alcohol, narcotics, or sedatives; use cautiously with major tranquilizers, antidepressants, and anticholinergics (drying agents); although 10–20 gms. are usually lethal, as little as 5 gms. have been fatal; interferes with anticoagulants, requiring careful monitoring by physician; not to be used by patients with glaucoma or porphyria; not recommended for children under 12

Table continues on next page

9.1 / *continued*

BRAND NAME(S)	GENERIC NAME (CHEMICAL CLASS)	USUAL THERA- PEUTIC DOSE	ACTIONS
LUMINAL STENTAL (Usually prescribed by generic name)	Phenobarbital (barbiturate)	100 mgs.	Decreased REM with REM rebound; hypnotic action lasts 6–10 hours; half life is 24–96 hours; wears off in 5–7 nights; reduces nocturnal awakenings

Comment: Because of its long half-life, it is the least desirable of the already undesirable barbiturate hypnotics.

NEMBUTAL	Pentobarbital (barbiturate)	100 mgs.	Decreased REM with REM rebound: hypnotic action lasts 3–6 hours; half-life is 21–42 hours; wears off in 5–7 nights; reduces nocturnal awakenings

Comment: Avoid. There are better hypnotics than barbiturates.

NOCTEC AQUA- CHLORAL (Usually prescribed by generic name)	Chloral hydrate (alcohol)	500–1,500 mgs.	Minimal effect on sleep stages; hypnotic action lasts 4– 6 hours; half-life of major active metabolite (by-product) is 8 hours; wears off in 5–7 nights; does not reduce nocturnal awakenings

Comment: Relatively safe and effective for occasional use; must not be taken with alcohol (Mickey Finn) or in more than the therapeutic dose.

SIDE EFFECTS	PRECAUTIONS
Same as with Amytal, except even greater likelihood of daytime grogginess	Same as with Amytal
Same as with Amytal	Same as with Amytal
Except for stomach irritation and allergic dermititis, there are few side effects; hangover and lethargy are uncommon; excitement and agitation occur rarely	Although toxic dose is 4–30 gms., it can be lethal at 4 gms.; never use more than 2 gms. in one night; should not be taken by patients with severe liver, kidney, or heart diseases; inhibits oral anticoagulants, requiring careful monitoring by doctor; *must not* be used with alcohol; can be habit forming

Table continues on next page

9.1 / *continued*

BRAND NAME(S)	GENERIC NAME (CHEMICAL CLASS)	USUAL THERA-PEUTIC DOSE	ACTIONS
NOLUDAR	Methyprylon (piperidinedione)	200–400 mgs.	Decreased REM with REM rebound; hypnotic action lasts 5–8 hours; half-life is 4 hours; wears off in 7 nights; effect on nocturnal awakenings is unknown

Comment: Relatively few studies on Noludar; its only advantage is a short half-life; otherwise, it's nothing special.

| PLACIDYL | Ethchlorvynol (alcohol) | 500–750 mgs. (500 mg. dose is preferable, especially in the elderly and the debilitated.) | Duration of efficacy and effects on sleep stages and on nocturnal awakenings are unknown; hypnotic action lasts 5 hours; half-life is 5–6 hours |

Comment: Too little is known about Placidyl. What is known suggests it's worth avoiding. Having a short half-life, it's better for initial insomnia than for middle insomnia.

SIDE EFFECTS	PRECAUTIONS
Few side effects have been reported; these include dizziness; nausea; vomiting; diarrhea; headache; mild hangover; skin rash; allergic reactions; may decrease platelets (for clotting) and white blood cells (for fighting infections); excitement and agitation occur rarely	Toxic dose is 6–27 gms.; do not use if allergic to Noludar; may cause psychological and physical dependency; must not be used by pregnant or nursing mothers, nor by patients with porphyria; should be taken cautiously by those with kidney and liver diseases; should not be used with alcohol, sedatives, or narcotics; continued use requires periodic blood counts; not recommended for children under 12
Nausea; vomiting; stomach upset; bitter taste; dizziness; low blood pressure; blurred vision; facial numbness; difficulty walking; mild hangover; allergic reactions including skin rash and urticaria. *Rare:* aggravates depression; decreased platelets (for clotting); jaundice (yellow skin and eyes); excitement and agitation; fainting; profound muscle weakness	Although 15-25 gms. are usually toxic, as low as 10–25 gms. has been lethal; should not be taken if allergic to Placidyl; must not be used by pregnant or nursing mothers; should not be taken by people with a tendency to depression; must not be used by patients with prophyria; use very cautiously with antidepressants, alcohol, sedatives, anticholinergics (e.g., Donnatal, Belladenal), Mellaril, or narcotics; should be used with caution by those with liver or kidney diseases; dizziness and difficulty walking can be reduced if Placidyl is taken along with food; psychological and physical dependency; may interfere with oral anticoagulants, requiring careful monitoring by physician

Table continues on next page

9.1 / *continued*

BRAND NAME(S)	GENERIC NAME (CHEMICAL CLASS)	USUAL THERA-PEUTIC DOSE	ACTIONS
QUAALUDE MEQUIN SOPOR PAREST *Comment:* No advantage for sleep induction. It produces a "high," making Quaalude a popular "street drug," but a dangerous and potentially addictive one.	Methaqualone (quinazolinone)	150–300 mgs. (150 mgs. is preferable, especially in the elderly and debilitated. Parest dose is 200–400 mgs.)	At 300 mgs. (but not 150 mgs.) get decreased REM with REM rebound; may decrease stage 4; hypnotic action lasts 6–8 hours; half-life is 1–4 hours; wears off in 5–7 nights; may decrease nocturnal awakenings
SECONAL *Comment:* Although it is one of the better barbiturates, all barbiturates should be avoided.	Secobarbital (barbiturate)	100 mgs. (preferably less in the elderly and debilitated)	Decreased REM with REM rebound; hypnotic action lasts 3–6 hours; half-life is 20–28 hours; wears off in 5–7 nights; decreases nocturnal awakenings
TRICLOS *Comment:* Hard to evaluate due to lack of research; chemically similar to the better-known and safer chloral hydrate (Noctec).	Triclofos (alcohol)	1,500 mgs.	Very few studies of its effects on sleep. Seems to affect sleep stages minimally; hypnotic action lasts 4–6 hours; half-life is 11 hours; wears off in 7 days, and possibly longer in the elderly; effects on nocturnal awakenings are unknown

SIDE EFFECTS	PRECAUTIONS
Headache; hangover; fatigue; dizziness; tingling sensations; stupor; dry mouth; no appetite; nausea; vomiting; stomach upset; diarrhea; sweating; allergic skin reactions; muscle weakness; confusion; chills; tremor; irritability; euphoria; impaired memory. *Rare:* Restlessness, anxiety; anemia; menstrual disturbances; nose bleeds	Toxic dose is 2.4–8 gms; 8 gms. can be lethal; do not take if previously allergic to Quaalude; beware of driving or operating machinery; do not take with alcohol, sedatives, or narcotics; psychological dependency very common; physical dependency also occurs; must be used in reduced doses by patients with liver diseases; effects on oral anticoagulants are unknown; not recommended for children
Same as with Amytal, except slightly less chance of daytime fatigue	Same as with Amytal
Headache; hangover; drowsiness; stomach upset; nausea; vomiting; staggering; poor muscle coordination; "gas"; "bad taste"; lightheadedness; allergic blood and skin reactions; nightmares; malaise; reduced white blood cells (for fighting infections); possibly confusion and excitement	Toxic dose is unknown; not to be taken by patients allergic to chloral hydrate or Triclos; not to be used by those with marked liver or kidney diseases; may cause psychological and physical dependency; not to be used by pregnant or nursing mothers; may cause (yellow) jaundice in newborns; not to be used with alcohol, narcotics, or sedatives; exercise caution while driving or operating machinery; should be used cautiously by patients with heart disease; blood counts should be done periodically; not recommended for children under 12

Table continues on next page

9.1 / *continued*

BRAND NAME(S)	GENERIC NAME (CHEMICAL CLASS)	USUAL THERAPEUTIC DOSE	ACTIONS
TUINAL	Secobarbital and amobarbital in equal parts (barbiturate)	50–100 mgs.	Same as with Amytal and Seconal

Comment: This combination drug does not have any advantages. Avoid. There are better hypnotics than barbiturates.

*1,000 mgs. = 1 gm.

Other Prescription Drugs Affecting Sleep

The ever-growing proliferation of medications has brought with it many drugs that profoundly influence sleep. Because these medications are not primarily intended to induce sleep, their soporific actions are actually side effects.

Table 9.2 lists the most frequently prescribed sleep-altering drugs. Most of these promote sleep, though a few prevent sleep. The table mentions their brand and generic names, along with the *therapeutic group* to which they belong. Within any single therapeutic group there are numerous medications that frequently, but not always, behave in nearly identical ways. A principal reason why there are so many drugs that act similarly is because the manufacturers usually exchange a few molecules, which then allows them to market a "new" drug.

If you're taking any of the drugs in Table 9.2, learn more about them. Although many of these medications can be quite effective in relieving specific symptoms, they also give rise to numerous side effects. In addition to asking your physician about the advantages and hazards of these drugs, I'd suggest consulting Goodman and Gilman's *The Pharma-*

SIDE EFFECTS	PRECAUTIONS
Same as with Amytal	Same as with Amytal

cological Basis of Therapeutics, fifth edition (New York: Macmillan, 1975) or Klein, Gittelman, Quitkin, and Rifkin's *Diagnosis and Drug Treatment of Psychiatric Disorders: Adults and Children,* second edition (Baltimore: Williams & Wilkins, 1980). The *Physicians' Desk Reference,* a widely available annual compendium of drugs, is also useful; but remember, the *PDR* is made up solely of data supplied by the drug companies.

Since there is a plethora of medications that affect sleep, the following information is a mere summary of their major purposes and significant effects on sleep, as well as a comment on their potential for psychological and physical dependency. These synopses are presented according to therapeutic groups. So if you're using any of the drugs in Table 9.2, note the name of its therapeutic group before you read these encapsulated remarks.

ANTIDEPRESSANTS These drugs are extremely useful for treating *severe* depressions (Chapter 10), a frequent cause of insomnia. Because most antidepressants, especially Elavil and Sinequan, are initially potent sleep inducers, they may usually be taken all at once at bedtime, thereby making the

9.2 / COMMONLY USED NONHYPNOTIC PRESCRIPTION DRUGS AFFECTING SLEEP

BRAND NAME	GENERIC NAME	THERAPEUTIC GROUP	COMMENTS
Antivert	meclizine	Antihistamine	
Ativan	lorazepam	Sedative	Benzodiazepine
Atarax	hydroxyzine	Sedative	
Aventyl	nortriptyline	Antidepressant	
Benadryl	diphenhydramine	Antihistamine	
Benzedrine	amphetamine	Stimulant	Dangerous
Chlor-Trimeton	chlorpheniramine	Antihistamine	In many cold tablets
Codeine*	codeine	Narcotic	Often combined with mild pain-killers (e.g., Tylenol, Empirin)
Coricidin	chlorpheniramine	Antihistamine	In many cold tablets
Cylert	pemoline	Stimulant	Only for hyper-active children
Demerol	meperidine	Narcotic	Highly addicting
Dexamyl	dextroampheta-mine and amo-barbital	Stimulant and Hypno-sedative	Dangerous
Dexedrine	dextroampheta-mine	Stimulant	Dangerous
Elavil	amitriptyline	Antidepressant	Very sedating
Etrafon	perphenazine and amitriptyline	Major Tranquil-izer and Antide-pressant	Avoid continued use
Equanil	meprobamate	Sedative	Relatively unsafe
Haldol	haloperidol	Major Tranquil-izer	
Librium	chlordiazepoxide	Sedative	Benzodiazepine
Mellaril	thioridazine	Major Tranquilizer	Quite sedating
Methadone*	methadone	Narcotic	Addictive
Miltown	meprobamate	Sedative	Relatively unsafe

BRAND NAME	GENERIC NAME	THERAPEUTIC GROUP	COMMENTS
Morphine*	morphine	Narcotic	Addictive
Nardil	phenelzine	Antidepressant	May disrupt sleep; use only on special diet
Ornade	chlorpheniramine	Antihistamine	Cold capsule
PBZ	tripelennamine	Antihistamine	
Percodan	oxycodone	Narcotic	Mildly addicting
Pertofrane	desipramine	Antidepressant	
Phenobarbital*	phenobarbital	Hypno-sedative	Barbiturate
Preludin	phenmetrazine	Stimulant	Dangerous
Prolixin	fluphenazine	Major Tranquilizer	
Ritalin	methylphenidate	Stimulant	Use cautiously
Ser-Ap-Es	reserpine	Major Tranquilizer	Mainly used for hypertension
Serax	oxazepam	Sedative	Benzodiazepine
Serpasil	reserpine	Major Tranquilizer	Mainly used for hypertension
Sinequan	doxepin	Antidepressant	Very sedating
Talwin	pentazocine	Narcotic	May cause insomnia
Taractan	chlorpromazine	Major Tranquilizer	Very sedating
Tenuate	diethylpropion	Stimulant	Use cautiously
Thorazine	chlorpromazine	Major Tranquilizer	Very sedating
Tofranil	imipramine	Antidepressant	
Tranxene	clorazepate	Sedative	Benzodiazepine
Triavil	perphenazine and amitriptyline	Major Tranquilizer and Antidepressant	Avoid continued use
Trilafon	perphenazine	Major Tranquilizer	
Valium	diazepam	Sedative	Benzodiazepine
Vistaril	hydroxyzine	Sedative	
Vivactil	protiptyline	Antidepressant	May cause insomnia

*These medications are usually prescribed by their generic names.

use of hypnotics superfluous. Although the soporific effects of antidepressants wear off within one or two weeks, after ten to fourteen days of treatment, the depression begins to lift and the insomnia ceases to exist.

Because antidepressants suppress REM, when you're removed from these drugs (but not before), sleeplessness and nightmares frequently occur. But these symptoms can be prevented if your doctor slowly tapers off the medication. Most antidepressants probably increase delta sleep, which might be an inadvertent blessing to the sleep-craving depressed patient. If antidepressants leave you groggy during the day, check with your physician.

Despite their soporific inclinations, on rare occasions antidepressants cause insomnia. When this happens, consult your doctor immediately.

Although antidepressants do not produce psychological or physical dependency, some patients with repeated depressions need to remain on these medications for a long time, or risk another serious depression.

ANTIHISTAMINES   Even though these medications are mainly intended to combat allergies, they also are frequently contained, though in small amounts, in over-the-counter sleep aids and cold remedies. Because grogginess can result from using antihistamines, when you take them be careful operating machinery, driving, crossing streets, playing sports, and so forth.

Although the more sedating antihistamines (Benadryl, PBZ) are often deliberately employed by physicians to hasten sleep, this practice is inadvisable. Antihistamines decrease REM and cause REM rebound. They do not, however, produce psychological or physical dependency.

MAJOR TRANQUILIZERS   These drugs (e.g., Thorazine, Haldol) differ from sedatives (e.g., Valium) in that they exert a specific antipsychotic action, whereas the latter produce only a generalized calming effect. Major tranquilizers are prescribed to obviate the hallucinations, delusions, disorganized speech, and peculiar behavior exhibited by patients suffering from mania (Chapter 10), schizophrenia, delirium, or "bad trips."

Unfortunately, many people who have none of these problems, but are merely nervous, often get placed on major tranquilizers for extended periods. Because using them steadily can produce bizarre irreversible movements of the face, limbs, and trunk, they must not be taken continuously by people whose *only* symptoms are anxiety, tension, or restlessness. If you've been using major tranquilizers for over a month, it's vital that you ask your doctor whether remaining on them is absolutely necessary. You may wish to get a second opinion.

Initially, very sedating major tranquilizers, such as Thorazine and Mellaril, can put and keep you asleep for an entire evening. Like antidepressants, major tranquilizers can usually be taken all in one dose at bedtime, thereby eliminating the need for hypnotics. Also like antidepressants, major tranquilizers lose their soporific properties within one or two weeks. By this time, however, the insomnia caused by schizophrenia or mania often disappears because the drug has begun to control the psychotic symptoms.

Major tranquilizers variously affect sleep stages, depending on the specific drug and dose being employed as well as the particular illness being treated. In psychologically healthy individuals, however, these medications generally have a nominal influence on sleep stages. But their numerous and often serious side effects preclude their being used appropriately as a sleeping pill, especially if this is done consistently. Major tranquilizers are not associated with psychological or physical dependency. Nevertheless, schizophrenic patients who stop taking their major tranquilizers often become psychotic again, requiring rehospitalization.

NARCOTICS If used appropriately, these medications are effective pain killers. Since narcotics and hypnotics both depress the central nervous system (i.e., the brain), they should not be taken concurrently, except during unusual circumstances, such as following an operation. Although for centuries narcotics were used to foster sleep, they should not be employed as sleeping pills, because they are addicting. What's more, single doses of morphine or heroin increase stage 1 sleep and nocturnal awakenings while decreasing REM and delta sleep. Addicts have diminished REM sleep.

Narcotics differ widely in their capacity to engender psychological and physical dependency. Discontinuing the use of some narcotics (e.g., morphine, heroin, Demerol) leads to serious withdrawal symptoms. By contrast, narcotics such as codeine, Percodan, and Talwin, create only mild withdrawal. But all narcotics can produce days and even months of insomnia, once the user stops taking them.

Although most narcotics sedate, Talwin can increase alertness; taking it within four to five hours of bedtime may make it difficult to fall asleep.

SEDATIVES   Sedatives are the children of hypnotics. They differ from hypnotics only in that they are consumed during the day and that they make you relaxed rather than sleepy. Otherwise they belong to the same family of drugs, the "hypno-sedatives"; they are chemically similar and influence your body in nearly identical ways. When taken in concert, sedatives amplify the effects of sleeping pills, and vice versa. Indeed, all of the hypnotics listed in Table 9.1 could function as sedatives, if used in smaller doses.

Although sedatives are taken while awake, they can disrupt sleep, because they can linger for twenty-four to forty-eight or more hours in the bloodstream. Sedatives of the benzodiazepine type, including Valium and Librium, the first and seventh most widely prescribed drugs in America, carry most of the hazards of, and affect sleep like, the benzodiazepine Dalmane. Barbiturate-type sedatives (and meprobamate) reduce REM, cause REM rebound, and produce the same side effects as do barbiturate hypnotics, such as Amytal (Table 9.1).

Sedatives produce psychological dependency and not infrequently physical dependency. As a rough guideline, the abrupt cessation of four times the normal dose of any continuously taken sedative can lead to a hypnoticlike withdrawal syndrome. *Consult your physician before stopping the use of these drugs.* Moreover, if you can avoid using sedatives, do so. You'll feel better for it, and certainly sleep better for it.

STIMULANTS These dangerous drugs (e.g., amphetamines) make it nearly impossible to sleep. Often called "uppers," these medications are frequently abused by students who wish to pull an "all-nighter" before writing an exam. This "chemical learning," however, usually backfires. Much of the information acquired under the influence of stimulants is subsequently forgotten. The sleep deprivation and agitation caused by stimulants will make it even harder to perform well on the test. Because stimulants produce euphoria, the student often overestimates his abilities and makes frequent mistakes.

Whether stimulants are taken by dieters trying to shed pounds, athletes attempting to get "hyped up" for the big game, truckers wishing to "fly" instead of drive, or teenagers yearning to be happy, their use invites disaster. Although it remains unclear if stimulants cause a serious physical dependency, they certainly lead to an overwhelming psychological one.

This psychological dependency is unfortunate, since low doses of stimulants do suppress appetite and improve athletic performance. Although stimulants increase athletic skills by only one to four percent, this slight edge could spell the difference between victory and defeat. Stimulants work not only by combating fatigue, but also by enhancing muscle strength and coordination, especially in well-rested players.

But if you're thinking of taking stimulants, don't start. Sleeplessness, agitation, tremulousness, irritability, violent outbursts, suspiciousness, paranoia, and psychosis are common side effects. For weeks, months, and even years after you stop taking the drug, you can feel perpetually exhausted and profoundly depressed and can easily regain whatever weight you lost, and more. Because stimulants are powerful REM suppressors, the REM rebound that ensues when use of them is discontinued causes fitful sleep and frequent nightmares.

They should be prescribed only for the treatment of hyperactive children and adults with sleep drunkenness (Chapter 8) or narcolepsy (Chapter 10). Otherwise, there are no well-documented medical indications for using stimulants. If your doctor is giving you "diet pills," ask him if they contain any stimulants. If they do, or if he skirts your question, switch doctors.

Although rarely used for legitimate medical purposes,* cocaine has become the choicest of stimulants. For a mere hundred dollars and the opportunity to go to jail, you can "snort" a few hours' worth of cocaine, get "high," and enjoy all the side effects produced by other stimulants. Steady cocaine use leads to REM suppression and rebound, sleeplessness, tolerance, and psychological, if not physical, dependency. Cocaine, however, is not the only recreational drug that affects sleep.

Recreational Drugs: Alcohol and Marijuana

By "recreational drugs" I mean all those chemicals that are principally taken for fun. Because two of them, alcohol and marijuana, have become so much a part of our culture, they are shaping the American way of life and sleep. About one-third of adult Americans drink alcoholic beverages at least once a week. Fifteen million Americans smoke at least one "joint" a day. To many, a party without alcohol or marijuana is a party worth avoiding. To many, sleep without alcohol or marijuana becomes elusive, if not impossible. For better or worse, recreational drugs are here to stay. Although they have been affecting sleep for centuries, only now, with the use of polysomnographic recordings, are we beginning to understand how these drugs modify sleep.

---

*Before he turned his attention to other matters, Sigmund Freud had made pioneering investigations along with Carl Koller on the use of cocaine as a topical anesthetic. More recently, cocaine has been incorporated into "Brompton's mixture," a concoction prescribed mainly in England to relieve the discomfort of dying patients.

Around 200 A.D. the Greek physician Galen noted that alcohol interfered with sleep. Although his explanation for why this occurred left something to be desired, his description of an alcohol-induced slumber was right on the mark. He observed that drinkers "stagger and are heavy in the head and even when force is applied they are unable to raise their eyelids; and owing to this heaviness they cannot sleep, being restless, turning from side to side and throwing themselves about and changing from one posture to another."

Unfortunately, his observations were ignored. After all, people had been drinking themselves to sleep long before Galen. Even today, "everybody" knows that alcohol helps you sleep. Well, "everybody" is wrong.

This misunderstanding undoubtedly arises from alcohol's initial capacity to induce sleep. What is not apparent, however, is that once you're asleep, the proportions of delta and especially of rapid-eye-movement sleep decline, while fluctuations between sleep stages accelerate. Not only is sleep unsatisfying, but, as Galen indicated, you spend most of the evening tossing and turning. Feeling exhausted the next day, you may be determined to get a good rest that evening. Because that alcohol will hasten the onset of sleep, the temptation to imbibe a nightcap becomes particularly appealing. After several days REM rebound ensues, producing nightmares, frequent nocturnal awakenings, and even greater daytime fatigue. You quickly discover that the terrifying dreams and middle insomnia are quelled by swilling another shot of booze. Because tolerance to the soporific effects of spirits develops rapidly, sipping an extra libation becomes necessary in order to doze off.

Once drinking becomes habitual, total sleep time actually increases. Unfortunately, this sleep is neither efficient nor refreshing. One of two patterns emerges. Either sleep becomes fragmented into numerous three- to four-hour segments, or nighttime sleep becomes supplemented by several daytime naps. Whichever pattern develops, light sleep prevails. Thus, even though you're sleeping more, you're enjoying it less.

If you're a heavy drinker who suddenly goes on the

wagon, you will be overwhelmed by REM rebound 90 to
100 percent of the day. Even though you're awake, frightening
dreams intrude into consciousness. You may start to misinterpret sounds and sights, and then be startled by auditory,
visual, and tactile hallucinations. You may see imaginary
mice or insects scurrying around the room. Disembodied
voices hurling hostile accusations may attack you from
every direction. Buzzing sounds, flashing lights, and darting
spots may bombard your mind. If you're lucky, this "alcoholic hallucinosis" will subside within forty-eight hours. If
you're not, delirium tremens or the "DTs" may set in three
to four days after your last drink. DTs have all the characteristics of an unrestrained withdrawal syndrome from hypnotics: insomnia, restlessness, rapid heart rate, sweating,
fever, agitation, confusion, disorientation, delusions, hallucinations, the sensation of insects crawling over your skin,
terror, and possibly convulsions. Without proper treatment,
10 to 15 percent of patients undergoing DTs die—usually
from respiratory collapse.

Many alcoholics who have survived DTs have told me
that they started drinking simply to get a good night's sleep.
Although other factors undoubtedly led to their alcoholism,
it is hardly uncommon to observe that yesterday's insomniac
becomes tomorrow's alcoholic.

Of course, not everybody who drinks becomes a lush.
But according to the National Institute of Alcohol Abuse
and Alcoholism, 36 percent of the adults who drink "can be
classified as either being problem drinkers or having potential problems with alcohol."

If you're unable to sleep without a drink, you're among
that 36 percent. No one likes to confess to a drinking
problem. But admitting this harsh truth to yourself is the
most crucial and often the hardest step to take in recovering
from alcoholism and the inadequate sleep that results from
it. If you require a nightcap or two in order to sleep, consult
your physician. If he slaps you on the back and tells you not
to worry, get another doctor. You also might look up
Alcoholics Anonymous (AA) in your telephone book and go
to a meeting. If you have an alcohol problem, I bet you that

any reason you'll devise for not visiting AA is a rationalization, and probably a lousy one at that. There are also meetings of Al-Anon for relatives of alcoholics.

There's nothing wrong with an occasional drink; but when you *require* a drink in order to sleep, you're treading on dangerous turf.

Unfortunately, you will be less able to predict the effects of marijuana or cannabis on sleep. Legal restrictions have made it difficult to carry out sufficient scientific investigations on marijuana. Furthermore, what is sold as marijuana is often contaminated with mind-altering chemicals, herbicides, or other toxic substances. Consequently the buyer has little idea what he is actually smoking and how it will influence his sleep.

Even if it's the real stuff, the effects of cannabis depend as much on the setting in which it is taken and on the expectations of the user as on the drug itself. If smoked in solitude, marijuana usually induces a state of relaxation and sleepiness. But when taken among friends, sleepiness is less pronounced. (This sleepiness contrasts with the arousal generated by LSD and other hallucinogens.) Scientific studies as well as the folklore of the drug culture suggest that novice users are often oblivious to marijuana, whereas repeaters usually experience the typical euphoria, hunger, time distortion, memory impairment, muscle incoordination, rapid heart rate, preoccupation with the present, floating sensation, lightheadedness, and difficulties in following through on complicated tasks. In other words, once "stoned" nothing happens, twice "stoned" everything happens. To explain this different response, one theory holds that you can experience a "high" only *after* marijuana has chemically primed your brain. A more likely hypothesis is that during your introduction to marijuana, you learn what to experience from others, and that therefore, the next time around you are prepared, willing, and able to enjoy it.

Adverse reactions to marijuana are more common among those who smoke because of peer pressure or who have negative expectations at the outset. "Panic attacks," characterized by an overwhelming sense of impending doom, account for 75 percent of all *acute* psychological difficulties that arise from marijuana smoking. These reactions usually last two to six hours, and infrequently for one to two days. (Psychoses are rare among marijuana smokers who do not have a previous history of serious mental illness.) These panic attacks occur in less than one percent of the students at university campuses where cannabis is frequently used. In contrast, 25 percent of the first-time smokers at a rural Southern college where marijuana use is considered deviant experienced panic attacks. Clearly the effects of marijuana depend more on the setting than on the drug itself.

Consequently, marijuana's effect on sleep appears to differ when it's studied in the laboratory from when it's experienced in the home. Even the relatively few investigations performed in laboratories have produced inconsistent, if not perplexing, results. Most laboratory studies have demonstrated that cannabis does not induce or maintain sleep, except in very high doses. In natural settings, however, marijuana sedates many people. But when chronic marijuana users refrain from smoking for twenty-four to thirty-six hours before sleeping in the laboratory, they fall asleep quicker.

Long-term marijuana use leads to small increases in sleep latency and in REM sleep, at least in the laboratory. There also is some evidence that smoking "grass" immediately before retiring diminishes delta sleep and increases stage 2 sleep. It is surprising, therefore, that when chronic, heavy smokers (averaging nine cigarettes a day for over ten years) do not take marijuana within two hours of bedtime, their sleep patterns do not change substantially that night.

The subjective effects of marijuana occur within minutes after marijuana is inhaled, peak at ten to thirty minutes, and subside after two to three hours. Cannabis is approximately three times more potent when smoked than when ingested. If swallowed, marijuana begins to produce its "high" between thirty to sixty minutes later; it peaks at two to three hours and gradually wears off by three to five hours.

Whether marijuana engenders psychological or physical dependency remains an open question. Although the data are inconclusive, it appears that a small proportion of users do become psychologically dependent on marijuana. A mild physical dependency may occur among heavy, long-term users, but not among conventional users. Indeed, experienced smokers claim that they develop a "reverse tolerance"; that is, they can obtain the same "high" by taking *less* marijuana. It is unknown whether this phenomenon is a genuine pharmacological property of the drug, a placebo response, a reflection of greater sophistication in efficiently inhaling the drug, or a convenient rationale for justifying its use. What is clear is that withdrawal symptoms do not emerge after stopping ordinary marijuana use. It should be noted, however, that abruptly terminating very heavy, long-term marijuana smoking can produce, after several days, irritability, restlessness, and insomnia.

Right now, millions of Americans are getting "stoned." And yet we know precious little about how this will influence their sleep tonight, their lives tomorrow, and their offspring for generations to come. I'm hopeful that, as the political and countercultural rhetoric abates, we'll be able to find some answers.

CHAPTER TEN

Detecting Sleep Disorders

It would be just as absurd to treat all types of sleeplessness identically as it would be to treat all types of fevers identically. If you had a temperature of 104 degrees, you'd surely want the doctor to find out its *specific* cause and give you its *specific* treatment. Yet when it comes to sleep problems, strategies for overcoming them are often pursued as if sleeplessness were a single entity.

If you're like most people, you may not want to believe that your sleep difficulties are due to anything besides "nerves" or "fate." You're especially unlikely to suspect that an underlying illness is responsible for them. It is sufficiently upsetting to go without sleep; to be told that you might have a specific sleep disorder on top of this may only compound your worries. It shouldn't. The detection of a specific cause for your problem may initially be disconcerting but may turn out to be a fortunate development. You would be able to obtain proper treatment, to stop aggravating your sleeplessness by employing useless if not harmful remedies, and to have the satisfaction of knowing that what troubles you is no longer a mystery. Let me illustrate.

Fortunately, Dan's job as a guard was at a teaching hospital. Ever since he was eighteen years old, he had suffered from "insomnia" and would nap several times a day. Although he didn't think that it had anything to do with insomnia, Dan also noticed that when he'd have a tense confrontation with someone, his muscles would become weak and he'd stagger around, at times collapsing to the floor. Dan assumed he was simply destined to be a terrible sleeper, and that he had to nap to "keep going." Though he wouldn't admit it to anybody, he felt he was a coward who feared getting angry; it seemed like the only plausible explanation for why he was unable to cope with anxiety-producing situations. These beliefs were reinforced by his physician. After completing a physical examination, this doctor told him that "nothing" was wrong and dashed off a prescription for hypnotics. (These pills made Dan so fatigued that he quickly stopped taking them.)

His boss, however, reached another conclusion. Watching Dan stumble, fall, and sleep at work, he maintained that Dan was either very lazy or very drunk. Dan knew he wasn't a drunk. But after years of dozing off in the wrong place, he became demoralized and blamed himself for "lacking motivation." Although Dan was given a warning, his symptoms persisted. Having lost two previous jobs for the same reasons, he expected to be fired any day. Then serendipity intervened. Because Dan worked in a teaching hospital, a sleep researcher happened to witness one of his wobbling episodes. After evaluating Dan in the sleep lab, the researcher's hunch was confirmed: Dan had *narcolepsy.* Treatment was begun and Dan's "insomnia," napping, and stumbling ceased.

Rather than being frightened by the diagnosis, he was relieved. "Of course, 'narcolepsy' sounds spooky, but so what? After all the self-doubt, embarrassment, and sleeplessness, I was actually thrilled to know that something *was* wrong. I'm not just a loafer, but a narcoleptic. Having this information has been an enormous boost to my ego. It's a comfort to realize that I don't need a 'shrink,' that I don't need to primal scream—although I often felt like screaming—and, best of all, that I won't be making a fool out of myself."

Like Dan, you might discover that your sleep problem *may* be due to an identifiable cause.

These specific sleep problems fall into two categories—primary and secondary. The *primary sleep disorders* are those in which the central features are disturbances of wakefulness or sleep, such as in narcolepsy and sleepwalking. *Secondary sleep disorders* are ones in which disruptions of sleep or wakefulness are auxiliary consequences of some other condition. Drug-induced insomnia (Chapter 9) is an example of a secondary sleep disorder. Psychological difficulties like depression or medical illnesses like asthma often produce insomnia, and therefore constitute other types of secondary sleep disorders.

Although employing the natural methods (Chapters 4–8) for overcoming insomnia will not aggravate sleep disorders, in most cases it will not alleviate them, either. Sleep disorders can be ameliorated only by the use of other approaches.

If you're to get a good night's sleep, it's important to see whether you have a specific sleep disorder. This chapter is intended (a) to alert you to the *possibility* that you have a sleep disorder, (b) to indicate if treatment would be helpful, and (c) to suggest the most appropriate way to confirm the diagnosis and to obtain treatment.

Narcolepsy

As a tennis player smashes a crosscourt backhand shot, he suddenly feels his legs giving out and plops to the ground. A mother gets angry at her five-year-old and slumps to the floor. Startled by a backfiring car, a teenager begins to wobble like a teetering top.

These episodes of sudden muscular weakness brought on by a strong emotion are all examples of *cataplexy,* the most characteristic symptom of narcolepsy. Cataplectic seizures may strike the narcoleptic once every other month or a hundred times a day. Whereas some patients experience only transitory weakness in a few muscles, others find that all their muscles (except those for eye and respiratory movements) give way. During a cataplectic attack the patient is fully awake and aware of what's going on around him.

The narcoleptic has a dilemma: If he ventilates his emotions, he risks becoming weak-kneed, falling down, and injuring himself. But if he suppresses his emotions, he puts himself into an emotional strait jacket. Struggling to control any laughter, tears, excitement, or anger, he may become more of a robot than a person.

The other major symptom of narcolepsy is the *sleep attack*—an overwhelming daytime sleepiness. Most narcoleptics are continually fighting off powerful urges to sleep. In mild cases, they remain awake, complaining only of "fatigue" or a "lack of energy." More often, however, they episodically fall asleep, usually for ten to fifteen minutes. Sleep attacks frequently occur at those boring times when most of us are tempted to doze off—watching a tedious movie, reclining on a couch, sitting through a dull lecture. Narcoleptics can also fall asleep at the most inopportune moments—while making love, driving a car, or robbing a bank. Dr. Dement tells of one patient who had a sleep attack while scuba diving twenty feet under water. To keep awake, narcoleptics often indulge in the consumption of coffee, cigarettes, and sweets.

Although cataplexy and sleep attacks are the most frequent symptoms of narcolepsy, the patient may also have *sleep paralysis* and *hypnogogic hallucinations*. On going to sleep or on waking up, the patient with sleep paralysis cannot move his body for several seconds or even minutes. While still able to breathe and move his eyes, he is frightened and frightens those around him. But if somebody touches him, the paralysis vanishes. At times, the narcoleptic can break the paralysis himself by vigorously moving first his eyes, then his eyelids, then his facial muscles, and so forth.

Just as he is about to fall asleep, the narcoleptic may have a vivid, often terrifying dream. Such a hypnogogic hallucination is frequently related to whatever was happening before he went to bed. For example, a Yale drama student had been rehearsing Hamlet's churchyard scene with the skull. While drifting asleep he saw his own skull being strangled by a cobra.

Hypnogogic hallucinations and sleep paralysis *by themselves* are experienced by normal individuals not suffering from narcolepsy. But when a person has *any two* of the syndrome's four symptoms—cataplexy, sleep attacks, sleep paralysis, and hypnogogic hallucinations—narcolepsy is the most likely diagnosis.

Sleep attacks often cause the narcoleptic to be awake at night. Thus, he paradoxically is awake when he wants to be asleep, but sleeps when he wants to be awake. He inevitably acquires a nickname—"sleepyhead," "lazy Tom," "slumbering Sam." Worse yet, it's dangerous to be a narcoleptic. Forty percent of these patients have one or more serious accidents as a result of having a sleep attack while driving. While rehearsing *West Side Story,* a dancer had a cataplectic seizure and ungracefully fell into the orchestra pit. Narcoleptics may also exhibit "automatic behaviors" —that is, they'll mechanically perform activities while in a trance. A patient may walk for miles, arrive at a destination, and then not have the foggiest idea why he went there in the first place.

Because narcolepsy is anything but a household word, it is more widely prevalent than you might expect. About 100,000 Americans have the illness. Narcolepsy often runs in families, and therefore might have a genetic basis. It most often begins when its victim is between ten and twenty years of age, but rarely after forty.

What had been puzzling about narcolepsy was why these four major symptoms should cluster at all. In 1962 the mystery was solved with the help of a polysomnograph. Whereas normally one drops off into NREM sleep and enters his first REM period seventy to eighty minutes later, the narcoleptic immediately falls into REM sleep. This finding explained the hypnogogic hallucinations that occur on going to bed; narcoleptics were dreaming as soon as they slept. Usually when people nap during the day, they first descend into NREM sleep. But when a sleep attack overcomes a narcoleptic, he dozes into REM. These uncontrollable bursts of REM also account for cataplexy and sleep paralysis. Except for eye and breathing movements, muscles are virtually paralyzed during REM. The four major symptoms of narcolepsy are thus produced by a sleep mechanism that has gone on a REM rampage. What initially triggers these excessive REM outbursts, however, is still unclear.

Treatment consists of counseling and medication. The illness is explained to the patient's family, especially to his children, who are likely to be terrified when seeing the cataplectic and sleep attacks. Five to ten evenly scheduled day time naps can minimize unexpected sleep attacks. Driving and swimming alone should be avoided. Patients may wish to join the self-help groups of the American Narcolepsy Association, 1139 Bush Street, Suite D, San Carlos, CA 94070, (415) 591–7979.

Medication is used to suppress unwanted REM intrusions. To counteract sleep attacks, the stimulant Ritalin (methylphenidate), keeps the patient alert and prevents REM from erupting into wakefulness. Antidepressant drugs, which also inhibit REM, prevent cataplexy. Although initially quite helpful, these medications begin to lose their effectiveness by the end of six months. Planned naps, however, can substantially reduce the reliance on medications, thereby allowing the narcoleptic to live pretty normally.

If you think you suffer from any two of narcolepsy's four cardinal symptoms, you owe it to yourself to consult the nearest sleep disorders clinic (Appendix A). The *only* way to confirm or refute the diagnosis is by having a single night polysomnographic recording. Because narcolepsy can expose you to life-threatening situations, if you suspect you may have it, find out for certain.

Sleep Apnea

If you're a heavy snorer *and* have trouble staying awake or not sleeping, you might have sleep apnea. Anthony Burgess wrote, ''Laugh and the world laughs with you;

snore and you sleep alone,'' but sleep apnea is no laughing matter. One study estimates that 1 to 5 percent of insomniacs are plagued by sleep apnea. It is the eeriest and most dangerous of the sleep disorders. If untreated, it can be fatal.

When these patients sleep, they stop breathing—hence the term "apnea," which refers to a temporary cessation of respiration. For unknown reasons, sleep triggers the brain to stop the diaphragm and rib muscles from operating or to collapse the windpipe. In either case, air is unable to pass through the lungs. After the sleeper has not breathed for 30 to 130 seconds, his body's oxygen becomes so depleted and its carbon dioxide so excessive, that he awakes suddenly, exhales forcefully, and snores loudly. He then quickly sinks back to sleep and this cycle starts all over again. This sequence can occur 300 to 500 times a night without the patient ever being aware of it. In most circumstances only his bedmate will notice the episodic gasping for air, the strident snoring, and the thrashing about that characterize sleep apnea.

But what does distress these patients is their unrelenting fatigue. Two-thirds of them suffer from excessive daytime and nighttime sleepiness; the other third complain of difficulties in getting to sleep and staying asleep. They often have high blood pressure, cardiac problems, and depression, and, as if that weren't enough, they're apt to sleepwalk. Frequently, they're obese—like the fat boy Joe in Dickens's *Pickwick Papers*. There an old gentleman describes him: "He's always asleep; goes on errands fast asleep and snores as he waits on tables."

Although Dickens had observed what was to become known as sleep apnea, physicians were until recently unaware of it. Sleep apnea was not recognized until 1965; only in the 1970s were its scope and seriousness investigated extensively. Consequently the disease has eluded wide attention even though its severe forms afflict at least 50,000 Americans. Because 80 to 95 percent of these patients are men, it's been estimated that half of all adult males with excessive daytime sleepiness *and* hypertension have sleep

apnea. If they also snore heavily, they are almost certain to have it.

The condition may also afflict children. Sleep apnea may be responsible for many cases of crib death, in which the infant suddenly dies without any trace of suffocation, distress, or illness. In the United States crib deaths—or, technically, the *sudden infant death syndrome*—claims 10,000 victims a year, making it the leading cause of death during the first six months of life. Older children with sleep apnea are constantly tired, tend to do poorly in school, misbehave frequently, wet their beds, get morning headaches, gain weight, and develop hypertension. Like their adult counterparts, they snore irregularly and vociferously.

If you snore and are chronically sleepy or have insomnia, you *must* be evaluated by the staff of a sleep disorders clinic. Only they have the expertise to diagnose this dangerous condition, identify its many subtypes, and recommend the best treatment. A great deal of harm has been inflicted on these patients by well-intentioned doctors who are unfamiliar with sleep apnea and prescribe hypnotics to help their insomnia. Because sleeping pills will depress an already malfunctioning respiratory system, death may ensue. Sleeping pills must be avoided.

If the patient is obese, massive weight loss can in mild cases alleviate symptoms. An experimental antidepressant drug (chlorimipramine), obtainable in a sleep disorders clinic, can provide short-term relief. Some children with sleep apnea can be helped by having their tonsils and adenoids removed.

If the condition is severe, and especially if it's life threatening, more drastic measures are required. To permit air to circulate through the lungs while sleeping, it may be necessary to have a tracheotomy, a small surgically created hole in the trachea (windpipe). During the day the patient closes the tracheotomy in order to speak normally. Before sleeping he opens it so that he can breathe. One or two days after this operation is performed, daytime sleepiness vanishes. Irregular heartbeats and hypertension subside within two to three months. Even the number and severity of the apneic attacks decline, suggesting that the lack of oxygen from inadequate breathing may aggravate the disease.

Don't be afraid to visit a sleep disorders clinic; the staff do not carry scalpels. A tracheotomy would be recommended only if *not* operating would lead to dire consequences. The decision to have a tracheotomy is *yours*. Avoiding the clinic will not make the condition vanish. For your own and for your family's well-being, if you think you might have sleep apnea, find out for sure by calling for an appointment.

Hypersomnia

When the trim Henry IV of France said, "Great eaters and great sleepers are incapable of anything else that is great," he was reflecting the old cultural bias still prevalent in our time, that sleepy people are lazy and stupid. This notion, however, is being challenged by contemporary sleep researchers. Persistent sleepiness is not a moral flaw but a medical symptom.

Hypersomnia means excessive daytime sleepiness that is *not caused by sleep loss*. Usually, the hypersomniac does not complain of sleeping too much, but rather of continued *susceptibility* to sleep. Although he obtains an adequate amount of sleep, he's constantly fighting the urge to get more. Whereas most of us take being alert for granted, the hypersomniac must struggle to stay awake. If he appears unmotivated or lacks that extra zip, it's not by choice. He deserves sympathy, not contempt.

Hypersomnia is not a disease but a symptom that stems from three principal diseases. Sixty-five percent of all hypersomniacs have narcolepsy, 10 to 15 percent have sleep apnea, and 5 to 10 percent are habitual hypnotic or stimulant abusers (Chapter 9).

In addition to these three major culprits, sleep drunkenness (Chapter 8) and disturbed circadian rhythms (Chapter 8) account for a small fraction of persistent hypersomnia. Episodic daytime sleepiness may accompany pregnancy, weight gain, hypothyroidism, and depression. And finally, there are a host of esoteric conditions that, in rare instances, give rise to hypersomnia.

Desperately seeking solutions, the hypersomniac often squanders thousands of dollars for medical checkups and laboratory tests. In a study of 235 hypersomniacs Drs. Christian Guilleminault and William Dement found that the average patient consulted at least three physicians over a period of ten to fifteen years; somewhere along the line his sleepiness was ascribed to "hypoglycemia," or low blood sugar. Although this condition may produce a rare case of excessive sleepiness, *not one* of these hypersomniacs had hypoglycemia. The vast majority had narcolepsy or sleep apnea, or they abused medications. But, the diagnosis of "hypoglycemia" still shines a beacon of false hope. If you're suffering from hypersomnia, the solution does not lie in faddish hypoglycemic diets, but in sleep clinics.

Kicking Legs (Nocturnal Myoclonus)

Almost everybody has had the occasional experience of suddenly kicking when falling asleep. When infrequent, these unintentional, reflexive movements are weird, but perfectly normal.

Nevertheless, as many as 10 percent of chronic insomniacs have kicking leg movements every twenty to forty seconds for several hours while asleep. These leg jerks can momentarily arouse the sleeper as often as 300 to 400 times a night. By morning he'll awake exhausted, even though he's unaware of the reason. Usually, only his spouse, who has in self-defense escaped to another bed, knows that he's been kicking and awakening most of the night.

This disorder is technically known as *nocturnal myoclonus* (i.e., *myo* = "muscle"; *clonus* = "spasm"). Although the cause of nocturnal myoclonus is unknown, several remedies can mask the symptom. Valium (diazepam) and Sansert (methysergide) can substantially reduce the frequency and intensity of these twitches. As a result, the sleeper awakes less often and feels more refreshed the next day. If you seek help for nocturnal myoclonus, you can speak to your physician; better yet, you can consult a sleep disorders clinic.

Restless Legs

Less commonly, people notice, on going to sleep, an uncomfortable, but not painful, creeping sensation deep within their calves, and occasionally in their thighs and feet. They describe this experience as follows: "It's as if my legs are full of worms"; "It feels like ants are running up and down my bones"; "It's like an internal itch." Although their legs are fidgety during the day, only when these patients lie in bed preparing for sleep do they become fully aware of their jittery calves. The feeling is so annoying that they will be unable to doze off without first "walking it off" for ten to twenty minutes. To drive this point home, the famed neurologist Dr. Thomas Willis wrote in 1695 that patients with this condition "are no more able to sleep, than if they were in a Place of the greatest Torture."

Patients with this "restless leg syndrome" invariably suffer from nocturnal myoclonus, although the reverse is rarely the case. Whereas patients with nocturnal myoclonus sleep fitfully through the night and complain of exhaustion, those with restless legs are bothered mainly by difficulties in falling asleep. At bedtime they feel compelled to walk or even to run around. Once they've done so, however, they're usually able to sleep restfully till morning and will awake refreshed.

Although the causes of most cases of the restless leg syndrome are unknown, iron, calcium, and vitamin E deficiencies are responsible for some of them. In one study 11 percent of pregnant women developed restless leg syndrome. Otherwise, men and women are affected equally.

If a nutritional problem exists, treatment is aimed at rectifying it. In severe cases Valium (diazepam), Percodan (oxycodone), or Tegretol (carbamazepine) can bring substantial relief. Daytime exercise accompanied by progressive relaxation (Chapter 5) or by meditation can also help.

If you suspect you have this condition, first check with your own physician. He may refer you to a neurologist or to a local sleep clinic.

Sleepwalking (Somnambulism)

A Detroit assembly-line worker on the night shift arrived home early at 2 A.M. and discovered that his wife and three children were having breakfast. When he entered the dining room to ask why they were up at this unholy hour, his family acted as if he weren't there, continued to eat, then rose from the table and mechanically sleepwalked back to bed. In 1878 a Scottish jury acquitted a man for killing his eighteen-year-old son because he had committed the murder while sleepwalking. Somnambulists have threaded their way along window ledges high above traffic, walked unperturbed across bustling freeways, and, with less success, tried walking on water. Sleepwalking thwarted the romance of a twenty-three-year-old Australian ingénue. While in a trance she tried to elope, but unfortunately her ladder was imaginary and she sleepwalked out of her second-story bedroom window.

Prior to Elizabethan times, sleepwalkers were assumed to be bewitched. Psychoanalysts also claim that sleepwalkers are "bewitched"—but by unconscious conflicts, especially ones involving the forbidden wish to snuggle into bed with the parent of the opposite sex. In *Macbeth* Shakespeare anticipated Freud by presenting a sleepwalker who was "bewitched" by psychological conflicts. Lurking behind a curtain awaiting the tormented queen on her nightly vigils, the gentlewoman and the doctor of physic marvel at the behavior and motivations of the sleepwalking Lady Macbeth.

GENTLEWOMAN: Since His Majesty went into the field, I have seen her rise from her bed, throw her nightgown

upon her, unlock her closet, take forth paper, fold it,
write upon't, read it, afterward seal it, and again return to
bed; yet all of this while in a most fast sleep.

DOCTOR: A great perturbation in nature, to receive at once the
benefit of sleep and do the effects of watching!

Lady Macbeth enters, trying to cleanse her guilt.

DOCTOR: You see, her eyes are open.

GENTLEWOMAN: Aye, but their sense is shut. . . .

LADY MACBETH: Out, damned spot!, Out, I say! . . .
What need we fear who knows it, when none can call our
power to account? Yet who would have thought the old
man to have had so much blood in him?

Although admitting, "This disease is beyond my practice,"
the doctor elaborates on the queen's psychodynamics and
offers the gentlewoman some therapeutic advice.

DOCTOR: . . . Unnatural deeds
Do breed unnatural troubles. Infected minds
To their deaf pillows will discharge their secrets.
More needs she the divine than the physician.
God, God forgive us all! Look after her;
Remove from her the means of all annoyance,
And still keep eyes upon her.

In this brief scene alone, Shakespeare the scientist makes
five acute observations. First, although in a trance, the
sleepwalker can perform relatively complicated tasks. Lady
Macbeth slips on a nightgown, opens a secret compartment,
and writes a letter. Second, her eyes are open. Third, the
sleepwalker behaves with selective attention and judgment;
the normally hyperalert Lady Macbeth is unaware that
people are spying on her and, with an uncharacteristic lack
of caution, verbally confesses her guilt. Fourth, *adult* sleepwalkers often have psychological problems. Fifth, the sleepwalker can physically harm himself, if not watched closely.

Today a "doctor of psychic" would amend a few of these
observations and correct other myths about sleepwalking.
Contrary to what you might expect, sleepwalkers are *not*

acting out their dreams. Somnambulism occurs only in delta, not REM, sleep. Moreover, because a sleepwalker typically gets up no more than once a night and does so within three hours after retiring, he usually forgets the entire episode by morning. Unlike Lady Macbeth, sleepwalkers generally mumble, and only a few words at that. Although an occasional one can perform extraordinary feats, most are clumsy; 72 and 33 percent of adults and children respectively injure themselves at least once. While sleepwalking, kids almost never harm anyone, whereas 28 percent of adults have at one time or another become violent. One of my sleepwalking patients clobbered his wife with a lamp. Another somnambulist set off an explosion by heating an open vodka bottle in his stove. Sleepwalkers have strolled out of windows and become black and blue by repeatedly bumping into furniture. After an elegant party, one somnambulist got up in the middle of the night and placed his expensive china in a clothes-washing machine.

Studies vary in their estimates of the incidence of sleepwalking. Between 1 to 15 percent of the population recall sleepwalking at least once during their lives. About 5 percent of college students claim they have walked in their sleep on one or more occasions. Four million Americans regularly sleepwalk. Because this condition runs in families, you can see entire families sleepwalking in unison.

The characteristics, seriousness, frequency, and treatment of sleepwalking vary according to the person's age. Somnambulistic symptoms in children usually begin at age six and taper off by age fourteen; adults typically start between ages eight and fifteen, and generally have three times more episodes a year than youngsters. Adult, as opposed to child, sleepwalkers are more likely to sleep talk (79 versus 67 percent), to experience night terrors (55 versus 14 percent), to endure nightmares (48 versus 33 percent), to report insomnia (28 versus 14 percent), to blame stress for their sleepwalking (80 versus 38 percent), and to stroll outside the house (55 versus 33 percent). Whereas twice as many boys sleepwalk as do girls, somnambulism equally affects men and women. So although 32 percent of adult and child sleepwalkers complain of bed-wetting, by and large, somnambulism is a much greater problem for grown-ups than for youngsters.

During an episode a sleepwalking kid will abruptly sit up, grunt a bit, and open his glassy eyes; he'll fail to see most of what's going on around him or to exercise critical judgment. If he remains in bed, the whole event generally lasts fifteen to thirty seconds. If he gets out of bed, his journey usually persists for five to thirty minutes.

About 10 to 15 percent of all children between the ages of five and twelve sleepwalk at least once. Persistent sleepwalking (one to four times a week) occurs in 1 to 6 percent of them. If propped up on their feet during stage 4, many children, whether spontaneous somnambulists or not, will go ahead and walk away. Ascribing psychological motives to a child's sleepwalking or sending him to a psychiatrist is therefore unwarranted; doing so only renders the child more self-conscious than he already is. Even without treatment of parental admonitions, almost all somnambulistic children automatically stop their sleepwalking within several years, especially by the time adolescence arrives. All of these facts suggest that sleepwalking is a strange but time-limited variant of a *normally* maturing nervous system. It should not occasion serious alarm, nor is it a disease.

Parents should take a "low-keyed" approach and reassure their child that he'll "grow out of this." In the meantime, as long as no harm is occurring, it's best to let the sleepwalker stroll about undisturbed. If left alone, he'll usually return to bed on his own. Don't startle the sleepwalker. When it's necessary to arouse him, do so by calmly and repeatedly calling (not yelling) his name until you've penetrated his trance. When he gives some indication of acknowledging your presence, reassure him that he's safe and gently guide his sleepwalking toward his bed. On rare occasions, however, these interventions further confuse and frighten the sleepwalker; if so, don't interrupt him unless he's in imminent danger. Parents can also protect their child by:

• Having him sleep on the ground floor so that he doesn't trip down the stairs or walk out of a window

• Having him sleep on the floor or in a sleeping bag so that he doesn't fall out of bed

• Removing dangerous objects from the entire house before their child goes to sleep

• Locking windows and, if the problem is severe, his door—keeping the keys with someone who, in an emergency, such as a fire, can unlock the door

• Tying a rope loosely around the child's waist and connecting it to the bed, for although most somnambulists quickly learn to untie the rope while sleepwalking, its tug may awaken him

All of these measures and the reasons for them should be discussed with the child in advance. Efforts aimed at minimizing his embarrassment are also essential. Drug treatment should be considered only when all these approaches have failed, and the child is in *constant* danger of injuring himself.

Sleepwalking in adults is unusual, more problematic, and often associated with psychiatric difficulties. Psychiatric consultation for adult, as opposed to child, sleepwalkers is advisable. Psychotherapy can reduce nocturnal journeys. Medications which diminish stage 4, such as Valium (diazepam), Dalmane (flurazepam), and Tofranil (imipramine) are sometimes helpful. Deep muscle relaxation through biofeedback and hypnosis has also been successful.

In addition, all the suggestions advanced above for assisting child sleepwalkers apply equally to adults. Two special notes, however, are particularly important for older somnambulists. Sleepwalkers can unlock closets and load firearms, which they've also used. Remove all weapons from your house. Finally, contrary to myth, it is *not* dangerous to waken a sleepwalker. Although he may be startled and confused, he will not become vicious or assaultive. Indeed, he'll be thankful that you cared enough to protect him.

Sleep Talking (Somniloquy)

W. H. Auden, the American poet, defined a professor as "one who talks in someone else's sleep." In this sense, sleep talkers are professors: Although they themselves are not bothered by their ramblings, those who must endure listening to them frequently are. Sleep talking may be annoying or amusing, but it is never pathological. Sleep talking is common; 20 percent of the population talk in their sleep.

Though sleep talking may occur anytime during the evening, 63 percent of it happens during stage 2 and 8 percent during stage 1. Because these are relatively light sleep stages, the sleep talker may have enough contact with his surroundings to engage in a conversation. But because he's still asleep, he's fairly suggestible, and therefore, his responses should be taken with a grain of salt.

Sleep talking during stage 4 occurs 20 percent of the time with adults, and more often with children. In contrast to those made during lighter sleep, stage 4 mumblings are often brief, incoherent, and boring. Because most sleep talking is a NREM activity, these utterances do not reflect dreams.

Ten percent of all sleep talking takes place during REM, where the sleeper will speak intensely about his dreams. Whereas you can converse with the NREM sleeptalker, you will find the REM speaker less cooperative; he's oblivious to his environment and too wrapped up in his dream to talk with you.

Sleep talking should not be treated. Benign quirks are not medical problems. If your mate's nocturnal verbiage bugs you, try using the remedies for overcoming distracting noises presented in Chapter 4. A final hint: One night, as my wife was babbling away during NREM sleep, I calmly asked her to be quiet. Lo and behold, she replied, "Okay" —and stopped talking. To my amazement, this simple and obvious method has worked ever since.

Nightmares and Night Terrors

A blood-curdling scream pierces the night air. Aaron's parents dash to his room and find him in a frozen panic. After comforting him, his mother asks what happened. Aaron doesn't know; he's just terrified. Eventually he calms down and returns to sleep. Although the following morning Aaron has forgotten the entire incident, his parents are still bewildered. Does Aaron have an emotional problem? Should they take him to the pediatrician? What actually frightened him? Will these "nightmares" recur? Are they to blame for their son's nocturnal horror? Indeed, for the 5 percent of parents who have children plagued by nightmares, these terrors of the night can be as scary to them as they are to their children.

At the outset, it's important to distinguish between nightmares and night terrors (Table 10.1). Aaron had a *night terror*, technically known as "pavor nocturnus" (night fear). Although they may occur anytime during childhood, night terrors are most frequently experienced by children between the ages of three and five, 2 to 5 percent of whom have them. These episodes usually erupt fifteen to thirty minutes after the child has gone to sleep. The longer he's been in NREM sleep before pavor nocturnus strikes, the more petrified he'll be when it does occur.

Night terrors erupt during stage 4 sleep and therefore are not the product of "bad dreams." It is possible to trigger night terrors in some children merely by awakening them or by buzzing an alarm while they're in stage 4. Why night terrors occur at all, however, is a puzzle, especially since the mind is practically a void during deep sleep. The child is unable to say what frightened him, or, for that matter, to say anything at all. At most, he may describe a solitary image—a ghost, a monster, a bogeyman. The child will awake screaming, moaning, crying, or gasping. Breathing rapidly, he will sit up with a wide-eyed stare. In extreme cases he'll tear through the house. His overwhelming panic, which often persists for ten to twenty minutes, generates a heart rate of

10.1/DIFFERENCES BETWEEN NIGHTMARES AND NIGHT TERRORS

CHARACTERISTICS	NIGHT TERRORS	NIGHTMARES
Time of onset	Within 60 minutes of falling asleep	Anytime, usually after 90 minutes of falling asleep
Sleep stage	4	REM
Anxiety	Severe	Moderate
Heart rate in children having attack	About 160–170 beats a minute	About 100–120 beats a minute
Associated symptoms	Sleepwalking and wetting	None
Recall immediately afterward	Little, usually none	Can describe the "bad dream"
Recall the next morning	None	May remember
Runs in families	Yes	No

TREATMENT	NIGHT TERRORS	NIGHTMARES
If episodic in children	None	None
If episodic in adults	Consult psychiatrist or psychologist. No medication	None
If persistent in children	Consult pediatrician or child psychiatrist; psychotherapy, play therapy. Valium?	Consult pediatrician, child psychiatrist or psychologist; parental counseling, psychotherapy, play therapy. No medication
If persistent in adults	Consult psychiatrist; psychotherapy. Valium, Tofranil	Consult psychiatrist or psychologist; psychotherapy or desensitization. No medication

up to 160 to 170 beats a minute—twice normal and faster than can be attained under almost any other stressful circumstance in life. Neither boxers in the heat of combat nor lovers at the height of ecstasy reach the astounding heart rate of the horror-stricken child with night terrors. Nevertheless, once hugged and reassured, the child will stop his sobbing, relax, and doze off. By morning he will not remember a thing.

Such a child may also be subject to sleepwalking and bed-wetting, which are, like night terrors, arousal disturbances from stage 4 sleep. What's more, since all three of these conditions run in families, a biological predisposition to experiencing them probably exists. Consequently, at least with adults, Drs. Anthony and Joyce Kales have postulated that those with more impaired stage-4-arousal mechanisms develop night terrors, whereas those with less impairment are prone to sleepwalking. The Kales have further suggested that personality traits also influence whether the physiologically cockeyed stage-4-arousal system produces night terrors or sleepwalking: those who *inwardly* direct aggression trigger the "fright and fight" responses of night terrors; perhaps those who *outwardly* direct aggression generate the "flight" responses of sleepwalking.

Nightmares, which are more common than night terrors, arise from dream (REM) sleep. They can occur anytime during the night, especially later on. Although he is upset, the child's anxiety is less severe than with night terrors. He usually can recount his "bad dreams." Younger children especially benefit from parental reassurance that helps them distinguish between the unreality of a dream and the reality of wakefulness. "Everybody, including mommy and daddy, occasionally have scary dreams. So do your friends, although they probably won't admit it. These are just dreams, they're not real. Dreams play tricks on us; they fool us into believing there are martians, when there really aren't any." Turning on the bedroom lights also enables the child to differentiate dreams from reality.

Genuine nightmares most often occur to children between

the ages of seven and ten. They are not associated with the sleepwalking or bed-wetting; nightmares do not run in families.

Although nightmares and night terrors most often haunt children, adults can also experience them. Whereas both symptoms usually arise sporadically, they can recur frequently. How you should respond to them depends on the circumstances.

Episodic night terrors and nightmares in children do *not* signify psychological problems. Psychiatric consultation is unnecessary; parental reassurance is. By taking your child's fright in stride, with concerned equanimity, you can convey that "everything is safe and under control." Nevertheless, don't tell your child that "nothing happened"—something did. Instead, reassure him that you know he's scared, but that things will be okay. If he had a nightmare, try suggesting what a ten-year-old said: "When I want to switch dreams, I simply blink my eyes and change the channel." A seven-year-old whose dreams were inhabited by bloodthirsty pirates was told to make friends with them. By simply talking about his dream in a low-keyed manner, you can show your child that because you're not afraid of it, he has no reason to be, either. Schoolchildren wish to identify with their parents; they seek to make their parents' attributes their own. Wanting to be like their parents is a healthy part of growing up. You can tell your child about one of your own nightmares and how you dealt with it. Showing your children how to cope with their nightmares helps them mature, feel secure, and experience love.

Persistent nightmares and night terrors are frequently associated with psychological problems. Consequently, you and your child should see a pediatrician or a child psychiatrist. Under most circumstances, affording your child all the reassurance mentioned above is also extremely useful. On occasion, however, children will fabricate nightmares (but not night terrors) just to get their parents' attention. Whether your child is doing so and, if so, why, is often difficult to discern. An outside expert can objectively make these assessments and provide you with practical guidelines for handling your specific situation. Although children outgrow them, if these symptoms are sufficiently paralyzing, short-term counseling, psychotherapy, or play therapy is frequently beneficial. Whereas Valium can reduce night terrors, medication should not be used to treat nightmares.

In adults occasional nightmares are normal; they are no cause for alarm. But *persistent* nightmares in adults deserve attention. They usually reflect some underlying emotional difficulty that can be rectified by consulting a psychiatrist or a psychologist.* Either psychotherapy or a behavior technique called *systematic desensitization* can substantially, if not totally, eliminate nightmares. But before any of these approaches is employed, it's essential to make sure that nightmares are not being caused by REM rebound associated with medication or alcohol use (Chapter 9). Removal from these REM-suppressing substances must precede any verbal therapy aimed at sweeping away nightmares.

Whether episodic or continual, night terrors in adults usually reflect some emotional disturbance. Unlike children with night terrors, adults with pavor nocturnus experience more daytime anxiety than grown-ups without them. Although night terrors are rare in adults, when they do occur, they can persist for years. One awakes feeling suffocated, entrapped, or squashed, as if a sumo wrestler had sat on one's chest. Psychotherapy can often bring about rapid improvement. Night terrors in adults can also be reduced by low doses of Valium, and, in contrast to those in children, by Tofranil.

Snoring

Protesting, "I'm not going to sleep with anybody who snores like that," a Silver Spring, Maryland, housewife

*Whereas a psychiatrist is a medical doctor who can prescribe medication and conduct psychotherapy, a psychologist is a Ph.D. who can provide psychotherapy but not medication.

whacked her husband over the head with a billy club. The case went to court, where the judge ruled that his snoring was not a justifiable defense and convicted her of assault and battery. Although snoring has been given as a *reason* for divorce, in none of the fifty states has it ever been a *grounds* for divorce. But if snoring can't spring you from marriage, it could spring you from jail. For swiping a night-club's loud speaker, Travis Zellis was sentenced for ninety days to a Cincinnati prison. Once he was in jail, however, his snoring so tormented the guards and inmates that the warden pleaded with and got the judge and probation officer to have Zellis released immediately.

Snoring stories abound because there are so many snorers. On any single night, one out of every six to eight men and women is gurgling, rasping, snorting, or hissing while asleep. Snoring is a great leveler; the sauve, dignified, wealthy, famous, and powerful snore as inelegantly as everyone else. A 1947 *Collier's* article claimed that twenty of thirty-two United States presidents snored, including Washington, both Adamses, Lincoln, Cleveland, Harding, Hoover, and FDR. Teddy Roosevelt's sibiliations were so annoying that when he was convalescing in a hospital, his fellow patients nearly instigated a rebellion. Beau Brummel, that quintessential ladies' man, snored, as did Plutarch, Lord Chesterfield, Winston Churchill, George II, and George IV, who boasted he was "the first gentleman of Europe." If you snore, don't be ashamed of it. You're in good company. Well, almost—Mussolini snored.

Snoring is caused by the rushing of air through the soft palate and the uvula, that stalactitelike soft tissue hanging down in the back of your throat. when this channel is constricted, breathing produces a vibrating noise similar to wind rustling through the reed on a baritone saxophone. This obstruction may be created by enlarged tonsils and adenoids, a deviated nasal septum, polyps, or allergically swollen mucous membranes. More often, however, there is no specific obstacle responsible for this nocturnal cacophony. Snoring typically occurs during stage 2 sleep, gets worse with advancing age, and usually happens when the open-mouthed sleeper lies on his back.

From an evolutionary perspective, the stentorian roar of the slumbering cave dweller may have had the advantage of frightening away predators. Today, however, snoring is a mere nuisance. Neither the health nor the sleep of the snorer is disturbed. As Mark Twain noted, "There ain't no way to find out why a snorer can't hear himself snore." Nevertheless, his bedmate can certainly be annoyed. Therefore, you might wish to try the following.

• *Humidify your bedroom.* Dry swollen mucous membranes can occlude your air passage and give rise to snoring.

• *Stop drinking and smoking.* Both activities can inflame, and therefore swell mucous membranes. Two to three months without drink or smoke is necessary to determine if abstention will substantially help.

• *Lose weight.* Because obese people are more apt to snore than thin ones, shedding pounds will reduce snoring.

• *Sleep on your side.* Some people snore only while dozing on their backs. Setting pillows under your back or using a body harness will prevent you from rolling over onto your back.

• *Use "snore balls."* During the Revolutionary War snoring soldiers had metal balls sewn into the backs of their sleeping garbs to stop them from lying on their backs. A tennis ball in a sock pinned to your pajamas or nightgown will serve the same purpose.

• *Beware of allergies.* Because any allergy can swell mucous membranes, hay-fever victims are more likely to snore during the ragweed season. Check to see if you're allergic to certain foods, pets, or fabrics.

• *Camouflage noise.* Wearing ear plugs, playing background music, and using other sound-disguising methods presented in Chapter 4 can help the snorer's spouse.

• *Stagger bedtimes.* To avoid being kept awake by your mate's snoring, you may wish to fall asleep before him.

• *Be wary of antisnoring devices.* Over 300 antisnoring

gadgets have been patented—none of them guaranteed to work. Chin straps, facial masks, orthodontic appliances, beauty caps, double-chin removers, and an array of weird head braces have all been designed to keep the mouth shut or to prevent the jaw from falling back. There also exist snoring amplifiers that selectively awaken the strident sleeper. Although some of these contraptions might help, don't count on it. Moreover, if your nasal passages are clogged, forcing your mouth to be closed will interfere with breathing.

• *Consult an ear, nose and throat (ENT) specialist.* Your physician can refer you to an ENT expert who will be best equipped to assess any structural obstruction, such as a crooked nasal septum or enlarged tonsils, which might be responsible for your snoring. Surgically correcting the blockade might be helpful, but advisable only in serious cases. An ENT specialist could also recommend nonsurgical antisnoring remedies.

• *Consider sleep apnea.* If you're an especially loud snorer, who is also a hypersomniac or an insomniac, consult a sleep disorders clinic to find out if you have sleep apnea.

Tooth Grinding (Bruxism)

Like snoring, tooth grinding can drive your bed partner to distraction. But unlike snoring, bruxism can be harmful to the "grinder." By wearing down your teeth, it can eventually lead to a lost tooth, an impaired bite, or damaged gums.

This annoying habit may occur while the person is awake or during any sleep stage. Most often, however, it begins after sleep has been nudged from NREM stages 3 and 4 to 1 and 2. Although nobody knows for sure why some people are compelled to grind their teeth, tension may play a factor.

If you're a tooth grinder, first see your dentist. He can equip you with rubber or preferably plastic tooth guards, which you insert at bedtime to protect your teeth from being worn down.

Daytime bruxism can be "unlearned" by biofeedback. In a United States Army study, by providing continual cues of

minute muscular activity to patients, biofeedback successfully treated 75 percent of thirty-three daytime tooth grind-
ers. How long this biofeedback training maintained its
effectiveness and whether it reduced nighttime bruxism is
unknown. Nevertheless, biofeedback treatment is promis-
ing. Your physician or the staff of a sleep disorders clinic
can tell you the best place to receive it. Make sure you see a
well-qualified professional. As is the case with many pop-
therapy fads, the biofeedback craze has spawned numerous
unskilled practitioners.

Secondary Sleep Disorders

All the vexations of sleep and wakefulness mentioned so
far in this chapter have been *primary sleep disorders;* that
is, ones in which the disturbances have been the *central*
feature of the problem. Another primary sleep disorder,
bed-wetting, will be discussed in the following chapter,
because it occurs almost exclusively during childhood.

Sleep is also frequently disrupted by psychiatric and
medical conditions. In these *secondary sleep disorders,*
insomnia, and occasionally hypersomnia, is only one among
many other and often more distressing symptoms. With
these diseases, attempts aimed solely at treating the sleep
problem without addressing the *total* illness will fail and
possibly backfire. Therefore, in your quest for a good
night's sleep, it's vital for you to spot and rectify a secondary
sleep disorder.

Three Faces of Depression

Everybody knows depression. A broken romance, a lost
job, or a loved one's death are obvious and nearly universal
causes for despondency. Nevertheless, the despair and sadness which follow these types of events inevitably wear off.
You're not quite the same person you were before, but for
the most part the wound heals, depression lifts, and life

goes on. These situational bouts with melancholia, however, are only one face of depression.

A second type of depression is experienced by people who are persistently glum. Their marriage is unsatisfying and their work unrewarding. Friends disappoint them. Fleeting crests of happiness are quickly drowned by waves of despondency. Enthusiasm for someone or something inevitably fades after a month or two. They "survive" more by habit than by desire. Life is drab, without purpose; its lack of vitality and richness haunts them with the fear that death will arrive before life has really begun. Psychiatrists say that these people have a "dysthymic disorder." Cynics claim they understand the human condition; romantics maintain that they appreciate that, in Victor Hugo's words, "melancholy is the pleasure of being sad." Others believe they're merely "indulging in self-pity" or "feeling sorry for themselves." Victims of such depression usually sleep longer than others, but their sleep is light and uninvigorating. Psychotherapy with a psychologist or psychiatrist can frequently enable those with dysthmic disorders to obtain a fresh and more joyful perspective on life.

A third type of depression differs significantly from the first two, both qualitatively and quantitatively. Psychiatrists have many names for it—"unipolar depression," "endogenous depression," "major depression." Although Sheilah, a forty-five-year-old woman, had been chronically unhappy, she suddenly developed a major depression, which she described as "a completely different feeling. I've never known what it means to be hopeless until now. My entire life is in shambles. The only reason my husband says he loves me is because he's trying to be kind. I'm a drag on everybody. Nothing, and I mean *nothing*, interests me. I once liked reading novels and seeing an occasional television show. But no more. As soon as I read a paragraph, my thoughts wander and I begin to worry that I'm losing my mind. Last night when everyone was trying to cheer me up, I just had to leave the room and cry. I don't even know why I was crying, except that they were being so nice and all I did was let them down. I'm sure I ruined their evening. Doctor, I can't go on like this.''

Although the nature of *major depression* varies from person to person, it is accompanied by a set of characteristic symptoms. Foremost among them are a profoundly depressed mood and/or a pervasive inability to experience interest or pleasure in normally enjoyable activities. One consistently feels sad, blue, worried, irritable, hopeless, helpless, and downhearted. Typically, these feelings are worse in the morning and subside slightly as the day proceeds. Laughter is virtually nonexistent. The patient also had many, but not necessarily all, of the following symptoms: poor appetite, unintentional weight loss, insomnia, loss of energy, agitation, slowed movements, decreased interest in sex, excessive feelings of self-reproach or guilt, an inability to concentrate or to think with one's usual degree of swiftness or decisiveness, and recurrent thoughts of death and suicide. Frequently, a vast array of physical symptoms or an excessive preoccupation with one's health can mask the depression.

Major depression may develop over a few days or weeks, but the subjection to a particularly stressful event may bring it on suddenly. Without treatment, major depression usually persists three to six months, but it may be longer, much longer. Once they've recovered, however, 80 percent of these patients feel like their normal selves. These depressions can begin at any time in life. Half of the people who develop major depression will never have another episode; the other half will ultimately have one or more bouts of depression. Studies indicate that approximately 18 to 23 percent of women and 8 to 11 percent of men will fall victim to major depression at some time during their lives. That means that about one out of every six people you know will eventually undergo this ordeal.

Both biological and psychological factors give rise to major depression. A relative deficiency of catecholamines and indoleamines—chemicals which transmit messages in the brain—play a major role in this type of depression. The identical psychological stress can trigger a major depression in a person who is prone to this chemical imbalance, but produce merely sadness in an individual whose biology makes him less susceptible to it. Whereas the loss of a job or the death of a loved one frequently precipitates a depression, major depressions very often come out of nowhere.

Insomnia is often one of the most distressing symptoms of depression. The despondent person may have difficulty falling asleep, or he may wake up in the middle of the night or arise early in the morning and be unable to return to sleep. Because patients typically feel worse in the morning, they are most apt to be troubled by sleeplessness near the end of the night. Whether or not their sleep is interrupted, depressed patients have less delta sleep, which compounds their daytime fatigue. Surprisingly, the *amount* of REM sleep is usually unchanged. But whereas normally the first dreaming episode of the evening occurs about seventy to eighty minutes after falling asleep, the patient with major depression enters his initial REM interval five to fifteen minutes after dozing off. When depression is treated with medication or electroconvulsive therapy, insomnia substantially abates within three to four days, even though the depressed mood does not lift for an additional week or two.

Until recently, there was no way of predicting if a particular depressed patient would respond favorably to a specific antidepressant drug until a thirty-day trial period of medication had elapsed. However, Dr. David Kupfer has shown that a positive clinical outcome with an antidepressant drug can be anticipated if the patient's initial REM period is delayed and the percentage of his total REM sleep is decreased after he has been on the medication for only two days. In any event, the relatively quick relief from insomnia is so gratifying that it often affords the depressed person his first ray of hope.

There exists excellent treatment for major depression. In most cases antidepressant medication, such as Tofranil (imipramine) or Elavil (amnitriptyline), will vanquish insomnia along with the other symptoms. If given all in one dose twenty minutes before "lights out," the antidepressants will help the patient doze off and make sleeping pills unnecessary.

In severe major depression, especially when the risk of suicide is substantial and immediate, electroconvulsive therapy (ECT) is the most effective available treatment. When introduced in the 1930s, ECT was often used indiscriminately. Patients with almost any psychiatric illness were frequently given twenty or more treatments. After receiving a brief electric current, they had a convulsion, which at times led to a fractured spine. These historical facts, coupled with a good deal of sensationalism, have given ECT a nasty reputation among the general public that it no longer deserves. Today, only six to ten ECT treatments are performed over a period of two to three weeks, almost exclusively on very depressed patients. With the modern procedure, the patient first receives a short-acting general anesthetic so that he is unaware of his subsequent convulsion. In fact, if you were to witness an ECT-induced seizure nowadays, you would see nothing but the patient's eyelids and toes twitching for about ten to fifteen seconds. Except for occasional and transient memory loss, ECT is a safe procedure that has proved to be a godsend, particularly for those most severely afflicted with depression.

Manic-Depressive Illness

Sleep problems also emerge in a fourth type of depression, that of manic-depressive illness. In many respects major depression and the depression of manic-depressive illness have identical characteristics. But approximately 6 percent of those who suffer from profound depressions experience at some time during their lives a manic episode— the exact opposite of depression. Whereas everybody has their good and bad periods, those with manic-depressive disorders go to extremes. When they're "high" or manic, they feel they're on top of the world; when they're glum, they plunge into the depths of despair. *Josh: My Up and Down, In and Out Life,* the autobiography of stage and Hollywood director Joshua Logan, aptly depicts his life with

manic-depressive illness. In between their periods of mania
and depression, patients with this disorder lead, like Logan,
highly productive lives.

When manic, these individuals are bursting with energy,
enthusiasm, and euphoria. Judgment and reason give way to
expansiveness and grandiosity. At our initial meeting, a
wealthy and normally subdued eighty-year-old manic woman wrote me a check for a million dollars. She added, "I
hope that's enough; there's plenty more where that came
from." (Stop wondering—I returned the check.) Manics
zealously pursue fantastic schemes. A UCLA sophomore
nearly reached Nikita Khruschev on the telephone to invite
him to the Rose Bowl. A scion of a wealthy family spent
$100,000 hiring architects, city planners, and lawyers, in
order to build a ninety-story edifice on one square foot of
land. Bustling with activity, manics are doing "twenty
things at once." To them, everything they do, see, produce,
or think is *the* best. In the space of ten minutes, a manic
Yale student showed me a thirty-page poem he'd just written—
"the greatest epic since Homer"; a new theory of relativity—
"I've discovered where Einstein went astray"; and a revised
constitution for the United States—"a landmark political
document." Speaking a mile a minute, manics have everybody in stitches, the way a fast-talking stand-up comic of
the Henny Youngman School gets a nightclub audience to
convulse with laughter. On a gloomy New Hampshire winter day, a huge Texan sauntered into the inpatient service of
the Dartmouth-Hitchcock Mental Health Center to "get a
check up"—and carrying two sets of golf clubs and an
enormous suitcase. Flashing a peace sign and singing "The
Yellow Rose of Texas," he mobilized within half an hour all
the patients, many of whom were depressed, and all the staff
members to sing along with him. People laugh with, not at,
the manic.

Unfortunately, their infectious humor and sublime ecstasy
eventually get out of control. Convinced that their way is
the *only* way, they become irritable, argumentative, viciously
inconsiderate, demanding, and at times assaultive. Once the
patients and staff got tired of singing, the Texan became

enraged. He told a despondent and very self-conscious plump teenager that she'd never marry because she was "too ugly." When most of the patients wanted to see the evening news telecast, he turned up the stereo so that nobody could hear. After politely being asked to lower the volume, he insisted in having his way and threatened to slug anybody who tried to stop him. As a manic Vermont truck driver said, "It's great to be high; I'm on cloud nine. I can conquer the world. But then things get out of hand, and I can be as nasty as hell."

The sleep patterns of manic-depressive individuals are mirror images of each other, depending on whether they are "high" or "low." Although they don't mind it, they sleep less than normally while manic. "Sleep is a waste of time; I've got too many important things to do," explained the energetic Yale student. Manics may not get to bed until two to three in the morning because they're "too busy." Whereas they'll sleep little while manic, they'll sleep excessively while depressed. Unlike the insomnia accompanying major depression, in this type of depression, the patient can easily spend ten to twelve hours sleeping, still be tired, and feel compelled to nap during the day. When manic, these people have a smaller proportion of REM; when depressed, their percentage of REM is greater than normal.

Very often insomnia and hypersomnia signal the onset of a manic or a depressive episode respectively. But some people may never develop the full-blown clinical picture. Instead, "mini-highs" lasting two to three weeks and "mini-lows" lasting one to three months will interrupt months or even years of relative equanimity. During these minor mood swings, the most prominent symptom may be insomnia or hypersomnia. In between these periods of aberrant sleep will be long stretches of normal sleep. It could be that these oscillating sleep patterns represent subdued forms of manic-depressive illness,* which might be helped by medication.

---

*There are many other reasons for fluctuating sleep habits, such as seasonal allergies, the flu, depressive reactions to the anniversary of a painful event, and altered work schedules.

The sleep disturbances as well as the other symptoms of manic-depressive illness can now be treated successfully with lithium, a mineral similar to common table salt. In smaller amounts, lithium occurs naturally in tap water. Although used for years throughout Europe, lithium became available to American physicians only in 1971. Lithium is not a panacea, but it has enabled the one million Americans burdened by manic-depressive illness to lead productive lives, whereas formerly their careers and families had been devastated by the disorder.

If you have symptoms of either major depression or manic-depressive illness, a consultation with a psychiatrist could be invaluable. Don't be embarrassed about seeing one. A fool is not someone with psychiatric problems, but someone who doesn't have the wisdom or the courage to seek help for them. Make sure that you feel comfortable with the psychiatrist and that he speaks plain English, not mumbo jumbo. If he appears to resent answering your questions, get another one. After all, you're paying him. At the same time, remember that psychiatrists are mortal; they cannot read minds, solve long-standing frustrations overnight, or provide the ultimate truth. What they can do is assess the nature of your problem, prescribe medication (if it is indicated), lend a sympathetic ear, and present a fresh perspective on what troubles you.

Obsessive-Compulsive Disorders

We're all obsessive-compulsive—at least to some extent; otherwise we'd never accomplish anything. But when obsessions and compulsions substantially interfere with getting things done, they constitute a disorder. If they plague you at bedtime, they'll plague your sleep as well.

Obsessions are intrusive, unwanted, and recurrent thoughts. The person knows it's silly to be preoccupied with these thoughts, but they persist nonetheless. Whenever Gary, a law student, left his apartment, he panicked at the thought that his camera might not be precisely flush against the right side of his bureau drawer. Gary was baffled. "I know it's trivial, even stupid, but I can't get it out of my mind." Compulsions are senseless, usually repetitive *deeds* which attempt to allay the anxiety unleashed by obsessions. Gary's compulsion was to return to his apartment three or four times daily just to make certain that his camera was properly situated. Patients with obsessive-compulsive disorders are not psychotic. The psychotic believes the irrational thoughts and actions are reasonable, the obsessive-compulsive does not.

Obsessions and compulsions can prevent sleep. Although he lived in a safe neighborhood, Gary was constantly worried that robbers would break into his apartment while he was asleep. Six or seven times a night, whenever he'd climb into bed, he felt compelled to check the lock on his door. "I know the door is locked, but something keeps driving me to take another look. When I resist the urge to check, my nerves become so rattled, that eventually I give in and look again. I'll stay up half the night worrying about this nonsense." Recurring obsessions are often about dirt or violence and lead to compulsive handwashing (as with Lady Macbeth), counting, checking, touching, or cleaning.

If you're plagued by obsessions and compulsions that interfere with sleep, the natural methods presented in Chapters 5–8 can be extremely useful. But if the symptoms still persist, don't put off seeing a psychologist or a psychiatrist. (Remember, not making a decision about consulting a therapist *is* a decision—it's a decision *not* to consult one.)

Heart Disease

It's ironic that sleep, which is so vital for the cardiac patient, may become his nemesis. If sleep were merely a uniformly quiescent interlude, it would continually afford the damaged heart the rest it needs. But although 75 percent of sleep is spent in the slow-motion physiology of NREM periods, the remainder of the night is devoted to REM sleep, a time of accelerated biological and especially cardiovascular activity. Blood pressure and pulse, heart, and respiratory rates increasing during REM. Dreams of intense anxiety are also of little help to the cardiac patient. Therefore, it is not surprising that heart attacks frequently occur at dawn when REM sleep predominates. One study revealed that 82 percent of nocturnal angina pectoris attacks happen during REM, even though REM constitutes only a quarter of all sleep.

If you have a heart condition, I'm not recommending insomnia for it. Sleep is vital, and REM sleep is unavoidable. What you can do, however, is prevent *unnecessary* and *excessive* REM activity in two ways. First, avoid hypnotics and sedatives, such as barbiturates, which produce REM rebound. If you need a drug to calm your nerves or to put you to sleep, use one that minimally alters REM, such as Valium, Dalmane, or chloral hydrate (Chapter 9). Second, if you're going to catch a nap, do so later in the day. Afternoon snoozes contain less REM than those taken in the morning.

More important than either of these suggestions is the caveat that you should not exaggerate the importance of this information about REM. REM does *not* stress the heart any more than does normal daytime exertion.

Ulcers

If you suffer from a (duodenal) ulcer, you're likely to awake in pain, especially from a dream. It doesn't matter whether the dream was a blissful odyssey or a nightmare; any REM period is apt to trigger pain. Whereas everybody else secretes less stomach acid while asleep, ulcer patients produce three to twenty times more acid while sleeping. This outpouring of acid peaks during REM and causes the nocturnal pain.

The ulcer victim thus faces a dilemma similar to that of the cardiac patient. Although both need sleep, this same sleep, particularly REM, aggravates their conditions. Consequently, if you have an ulcer, avoid morning naps and drugs that generate REM rebound.

Asthma

Nighttime is notoriously the worst time for the asthmatic. Wheezing, coughing, and shortness of breath readily interrupt his sleep. Although these nocturnal attacks may occur at any time for adults, they are less apt to erupt during deep sleep. Childhood asthmatic attacks during stage 4 are virtually nonexistent. Delta sleep seems to "protect" the asthmatic. Since there is less deep sleep during the latter half of the night, it is then that asthmatic attacks occur most often.

The asthmatic is likely to slumber peacefully through the evening without having an attack if he increases his stage 4 sleep. And the best way to do so is by exercising daily as described in Chapter 4. Keep in mind, however, that overdoing it can bring on wheezing; so exercise moderately and only after checking with your physician. It's also advisable to refrain from taking hypnotics that reduce delta sleep, such as Dalmane.

Thyroid Problems

The thyroid gland, which appears as a fat *I* lounging on its side in front of your throat, produces a hormone that stimulates your metabolism. The more hormone, the faster your metabolism, and vice versa. A goiter is an enlarged thyroid. Depending on what causes the goiter, thyroid hormone may be elevated, diminished, or normal. The condition resulting from excessive thyroid hormone is called "hyperthyroidism"; a depleted amount of thyroid hormone gives rise to "hypothyroidism."

Accompanying the accelerated metabolic rate of *hyperthyroidism* is short, fragmented sleep. Stage 4 can jump from its usual 15 percent of sleep to as much as 70 percent. Although hyperthyroidism is readily treatable, if it has persisted for a while, it may take up to a year for sleep to return to normal.

Besides insomnia, hyperthyroidism causes a fine tremor,

nervousness, excessive sweating, palpitations, and unintentional weight loss. When everybody else says the temperature in a room is just fine, these patients consistently feel it's too warm. If you have insomnia along with these other symptoms, consult your physician.

Hypothyroidism prolongs sleep but diminishes the proportion of stage 4. The patient constantly feels tired and moves sluggishly. When everyone is warm, the hypothyroid patient feels cold. With treatment, sleep very gradually returns to normal.

Because of the recent "natural healing" craze, hormone disturbances are now being attributed to just about everything. Sleepiness and a lack of pep are fashionably ascribed to hypothyroidism; nervousness and insomnia are conveniently blamed on hyperthyroidism. Thyroid problems are common, but not *that* common. Before leaping to the conclusion that your thyroid causes everything that ails you, make sure there's solid medical evidence to substantiate your hunch.

Epilepsy

In order to diagnose epilepsy, physicians often perform an EEG while the patient is asleep. Sleep frequently provokes seizures in those who already have epilepsy. Indeed epileptics, whether adults or children, are more likely to suffer an attack when tired or asleep. In one study of 645 epileptics, 6 percent of them, whether adults or children, had their seizures *exclusively* while sleeping.

Violent, uncontrollable shaking is what an epileptic seizure usually brings to our minds. But epilepsy takes many other less common forms, such as momentary lapses of consciousness and trancelike movements. Since epilepsy occurs in many unfamiliar ways, a person may awake in the middle of the night or complain of poor sleep without realizing that he was having a seizure. Of course, the odds that your insomnia is due to epilepsy are slim. You should, however, see your doctor (or a neurologist) in order to have the possibility of epilepsy checked out, if you (a) episodically wet your bed, (b) repeatedly awake with a bitten tongue or unexplained bruises, (c) have blood on your pillow for no apparent reason, or (d) are described by someone else as exhibiting seizurelike behavior.

Because epilepsy is a disease of the brain, any medication that affects the brain—including hypnotics, sedatives, antidepressants, tranquilizers, and narcotics—can trigger a convulsion. If you have epilepsy, don't take or change the dose of *any* of these drugs until you've received your physician's explicit approval. Treatment of epilepsy with anticonvulsant drugs usually controls the seizures which then restores sleep to normal. Once this occurs, following good sleep habits (Chapter 4) will reduce the likelihood of having fatigue-induced convulsions. Adopting a regular sleep schedule (Chapter 4) is especially important for the epileptic, because altered circadian rhythms (Chapter 8) can also instigate a seizure. Although the epileptic carries heavy emotional and physical burdens, careful attention to sleep can go a long way toward lightening them.

Two Caveats

I'm concerned that some of you, on reading about these specific sleep disorders, will contract "medical-students' disease"—an "affliction" whereby you "catch" every disease you read about. Worrying about an illness, whether it exists or not, can at times be as distressing as the illness itself. If you're likely to get "medical-students' disease," recognize it and place your fears into a reasonable perspective.

My other worry is that, sensing you have one of these specific sleep disorders, you'll not do anything about it. Whether it stems from laziness or fear of receiving "bad news," the reluctance to consult a professional is understandable, but ultimately self-defeating. The disturbing uncertainty that comes from wondering whether you have a particular problem is not avoided by avoiding help. It only escalates. Getting a consultation provides you with peace of mind, which, by itself, enables you to sleep.

CHAPTER ELEVEN

Helping Children Sleep

If you can't sleep, you suffer alone; if your child can't sleep, everybody suffers. When your newborn arrives home, you're suddenly up half the night. As he wails from his crib, you'll be torn between letting him cry and comforting him. Head banging, sleepwalking, and bed-wetting may keep the entire family awake. While he grows up, you'll lose sleep over his going to bed too late and getting up too early. His nightmares will give you nightmares; but his dreams will become your dreams.

Although all of your child's sleep problems and all of your sleepless nights will not happen at once, they *will* occur. A survey of forty-eight mothers of two-year-olds revealed that 27 percent of them currently worried about their child's sleep and that an additional 19 percent admitted to having previously had such concerns. Thus, in less than three years of being a parent, nearly half of you will be distressed by your child's erratic sleep. By the time adolescence arrives, nearly all parents will have coped with some type of major childhood sleep problem.

One complicating aspect of helping your child sleep is that his sleep requirements, patterns, and difficulties, unlike an adult's, continually change. So just when you've learned to deal with one problem another arises.

Another dilemma you face is contending with conflicting advice. When confronted with a problem, you'll receive a dozen contradictory suggestions from relatives and friends— all convinced that their answer is the *only* answer. But there is no "right" answer. If there were, theories of child rearing would not change like Paris fashions. When faced with conflicting advice, don't become immobilized by engaging in a never-ending quest for *the* correct answer—it doesn't exist. Every remedy has its pluses and minuses. Recognizing that no solution is perfect, you simply have to choose what strikes you as the best possible approach.

This principle also applies to advice offered by the "experts," myself included. For when it comes to your child, you are the expert. I can speak only about children in general; you alone know about your child in particular. However sensible my advice may seem, to implement it, you have to agree with it, feel comfortable acting on it, and, frankly, take responsibility for it. The value of my recommendations does not rest with how useful they are for others, but with how successful they are for you.

How Much Sleep Does Your Child Need?

Childhood sleep requirements vary enormously. During the first week of life, two-thirds of all newborns slumber between fourteen and eighteen hours a day. This means that one out of three infants snoozes *outside* the normal range. So if your new arrival sleeps a mere twelve hours, don't be alarmed. It's normal to be abnormal. Although the sleep needs of children steadily decline as they grow older, a tremendous range in sleep duration persists.

Table 11.1 shows you how long the typical child sleeps; it does not tell you how long *your* child should sleep. This table is a useful reference; it is not a divine dictum. Every child and his sleep are unique.

Nonetheless, many parents are upset when their child, God forbid, sleeps less than what the "experts" indicate. Although parents of short sleepers often fear for the health of their child, this fear is seldom warranted. Almost always, the briefly sleeping child is an efficient sleeper, not a poor sleeper. Indeed, many short-sleeping children are often physically and emotionally healthier than long-sleeping ones.

Of course, there are times when your child's sleep is *not* sufficient. Brief sleep by itself is nothing to worry about, but if it is followed by excessive daytime fussiness, irritability, fatigue, or whining, your youngster *may* require more sleep than he's getting. This is especially true if all at once he starts sleeping a few hours less than what is normal for him.

Because there are many other causes for an excessively fussy child—a tense parent-child relationship, poor feeding, overstimulation, and illness—it may be hard to evaluate the

11.1/SLEEP IN CHILDREN (in hours)

AGE	TOTAL SLEEP TIME	RANGE*
1 week	16.3	14–18
2 weeks	16.2	14–18
4 weeks	15.1	13–17
8 weeks	15.0	14–17
12 weeks	15.0	13–17
16 weeks	14.7	13–16
20 weeks	14.2	12.5–16
24 weeks	13.8	12–15.6
6 months	13.7	11.7–15.5
1 year	13.2	11.4–15
2 years	12.5	11–13.3
3 years	11.5	10.5–12.5
4 years	11.3	10.5–12
5 years	11.0	10–11.5
6 years	11.0	10–11.5
10 years	10.0	9–11
15 years	9.0	7–11
16 years	8.0	6.5–11

*Two-thirds of children fall within this range.

extent to which inadequate sleep contributes to his irritability. If sleep loss is not the obvious culprit, you should check with your pediatrician.

But when he's not unusually cranky or tired during the day, he normally *is* obtaining enough sleep. If you ask, "How long should my child sleep?" I'll echo Dr. Wilse Webb's standard reply: "I can't answer you, but your child can." In other words, with the exceptions noted above, how long your child sleeps is how long your child should sleep. Coaxing him to sleep longer than he naturally does will neither increase his sleep nor foster a favorable attitude toward sleep.

Mini-Owls and Mini-Larks

The variability found in how long children sleep also extends to *when* they sleep. Some kids nap, others don't. Like adults, some children are "owls" while others are "larks" (Chapter 8). Whereas larks spring out of bed and are raring to go at ungodly hours, owls slumber late into the morning and come to life only in the afternoon.

Schools are designed for larks, not owls. By the time the lark begins his first class, he's wide awake and fully able to learn. In contrast, the owl may oversleep and arrive at school late. Even if he stumbles into class on time, he sits bleary-eyed, and may not be able to learn optimally until after lunch. In the morning, his teachers may incorrectly attribute his lethargy to lack of interest, to stupidity, or to "staying up all night." (Although the extent of the problem has not been documented accurately, it's frightening to speculate how often this misunderstanding occurs.) If your child is hard to arouse, mopes around in the morning like a "zombie," and has his greatest difficulties in earlier classes, his scholastic problems may not be due to a lack of sleep or motivation. Instead, he may be an "owl." Granted, there are many other reasons for learning difficulties. But if your child is an owl, this fact should be discussed with his teachers. It's possible that his schedule could be rearranged so that he can take his more taxing subjects in the afternoon.

Being an owl can affect not only your child's education, but also his self-esteem. A child may be embarrassed that in the morning he's not as proficient as his friends. A Little League baseball teammate of mine usually struck out in morning games, but slugged home runs in afternoon games. Since most of our games occurred in the morning, my buddy consistently felt he had "clutched" and let down his teammates. He had, but not for the reason he and everyone else thought. In retrospect, I think he probably was an owl who was the unwitting victim of an abnormal biorhythm.

Just as with adults, altered circadian rhythms produce mini-owls and mini-larks. Circadian rhythms are largely determined biologically and cannot be changed very much. But they can be nudged. It may require only a minor shift in a circadian pattern for an owlet to fly on time with the rest of the flock. The methods for identifying and rectifying altered biorhythms that are presented in Chapter 8 apply as well to children as to adults.

Nocturnal Nemeses

You're alone and trapped in a room. Except for a glimmer of moonlight sneaking in through the rear window, all is darkness. Suddenly an ominous shadow leaps from the ceiling to the wall and then just as suddenly vanishes. Lying in bed, you wonder where the shadow could have gone. Your curiosity turns to panic, when for no apparent reason your right leg twitches. Perhaps the shadow crept inside your leg. Eventually your mind wanders to indecipherable mumblings from the room below. You're convinced that "they"—those who placed you into the room—are talking about you. As you become sleepier, you contemplate what "they" have in store for you. The next thing you know is that a tarantula is about to sting you.

You might dismiss this scene as lacking believability, but to some children who are falling asleep, it can be terribly real. Children understand, experience, and perceive sleep differently than adults.

For many youngsters, going to sleep is a harrowing ordeal. At the outset, they may sense, at times accurately, that their parents want them in bed so that they'll be out of the way. Their festering resentment may spill over into the scary fantasies unleashed by darkness. As if confined to a house haunted by intimidating dreams, shadows, and noises, they hide under the covers. Apt to confuse sleeping with dying, they may fear that they will never awake after going to sleep. Routine but unfamiliar bodily sensations petrify them. Jerky leg movements feel weird. When they are half-asleep, the common sensation of falling spooks them. Yet just when all their fears of darkness and sleep are most frightening, they are separated from the adults they love and need.

Kids episodically blend fantasy with reality. Those aged three to six in particular are apt to view a shadow not merely as an image produced by the interception of light rays, but as an organic essence endowed with mystical powers. Remember how relieved Peter Pan was on rediscovering his "very own shadow"? When a shadow disappears, it is only natural to ask where it went.

Growing up entails comprehending the relationship between cause and effect. But whereas adults do so with logical thinking, younger children often employ magical thinking. Although you know that a reflexive kick made on going to bed is perfectly normal (Chapter 10), your child may attribute his nocturnal twitch to a recently vanished shadow that has invaded his body.

To a small child, dreams are reality. When an adult awakens from a nightmare he knows it was only a dream. But that tarantula is as real to a child as it would be to you if it was actually crawling up your throat.

Younger children are egocentric; they tend to relate events to themselves. Sensory experiences are assigned personal meanings. To the child, honking automobiles convey secret codes; shadows are friends or sorcerers; street lights are magical rays from outer space. If a child faintly hears his parents conversing downstairs, he assumes they're talking about him and that it must be serious; otherwise, why would they be whispering?

Their episodic blending of reality with fantasy, their propensity for magical thinking, and their egocentricity are accentuated by darkness. Children develop their knowledge of things largely by seeing them. But in darkness sight is nearly obliterated, and the child must fall back on his imagination. Monsters and robots, hobgoblins and dinosaurs are the stuff of a child's imagination; in the dark they spring to life. In the absence of external stimuli, internal stimuli prevail.

Although a child's fear of the dark commonly exists from the ages of two to seven, it is greatest around three and four. But for older children, the prospect of sleep, and sleep itself, generates other concerns. Most boys (and too many adults) fail to realize that erections occur naturally during sleep. But whereas an adult will take this in stride, a child, especially from the ages of six to twelve, may attribute his erections to sinful thoughts, deeds, or dreams. Then too, after the age of ten, some children have sleep paralysis; for a few seconds on waking up they'll be unable to move their muscles. As explained in Chapter 10, sleep paralysis, by itself, is a transient and normal phenomenon. To the unsuspecting child, however, it can be a terrifying experience.

Of course, not all children are terror-stricken while falling asleep. But many are—probably more than you might imagine. A seven-year-old confided to me, "I'm scared of the dark, but I don't want to tell my friends or even my parents. They'll think I'm a sissy." The nemeses of the night can panic even the most stout-hearted of children. So the next time you send your child to bed, think about what it means to sleep, not to your mind, but to his.

Childhood Temperament and Parental Style

Parents often comment that although one of their children was easy to manage, another was impossible. In trying to account for these differences, they might wonder if their children were born or raised differently. Indeed, infants are biologically endowed with varying *temperaments,* which persist until they reach the age of two and often until they begin school. Research has shown that infants can be classified into three groups, according to temperament: the "easy," the "difficult," and the "slow to warm up."

A major study conducted in New York City revealed that 40 percent of the infants are "easy" children. Characteristically they are calm, sociable, attentive, and cheerful; they sleep regularly and quietly. "Difficult" children, constituting 10 percent of the group, feed and sleep erratically, withdraw from strangers and new experiences, and are readily frustrated, fussy, and inattentive. Fifteen percent of the infants are "slow to warm up." They lie quietly while asleep, withdraw from novel stimuli, and are relatively inactive, passive, shy, subdued, and sad. But with continued unobtrusive parental contact, they become more engaged. (The remaining 35 percent have some of the characteristics of infants in all three groups.) The "easy" child is simple to love; the "difficult" child is taxing; the "slow to warm up" child requires patience.

Parents also differ in their ways of coping with children of varying temperaments. The question of whether a particular child and his parents are "good" or "bad" is less important than whether the youngster's temperament meshes favorably with his parents' particular *style* of child rearing. Some parents are simply more adept at handling the "difficult" child. The same parent, however, might have more problems in contending with the "slow to warm up" child. In contrast, another parent will display great skill with the "slow to warm up" child but have significant trouble in coping with the "difficult" child. Therefore, whether the child thrives depends substantially on the existence of a proper match-up between the parents' style of rearing and the child's temperament.

How easily your baby goes to bed and sleeps is also determined in part by your child's natural temperament and your reactions to it. Consequently, there is no single way for you to approach your child's sleep problems.

Getting Your Child to Sleep

In many homes the battle of the bed rages nightly. Intimidation, manipulation, coaxing, bargaining, threats, and punishment are the weapons of combat. Though the conflict often begins as a mere struggle over getting your child to sleep, it can mushroom into a clash of wills to determine who's the general and who's the buck private. In the end everyone loses. So try to avoid the battle of the bed.

When you tell your child to go to bed, know why you're doing so. Maybe you feel he needs to sleep. Maybe you want some peace and quiet. Maybe it's a punishment. Maybe it's all of the above. Whatever your reason, recognize what it is, because your subsequent strategy depends on it.

Conjuring up extraneous reasons for sending your child to bed can taint his feelings about sleep. It's fine for you to have a tranquil interlude, but you should not pretend that your child needs to sleep. Not only do kids usually see through this deception, but they may begin to view sleep as something you do when your parents want to get rid of you. Instead of sending your child to bed if you want some peace and quiet, tell him to read a comic book, memorize a dictionary, or paint a masterpiece. But don't act as if he needed to sleep when, in truth, all you want is some well-deserved privacy.

Similarly, don't use sleep as a punishment. Disciplining your child by ordering him to bed will merely generate a disdain for sleep. Many adults who dread going to bed recall that as children they were threatened with sleep if they were "naughty." Sleep should be a pleasure, not a punishment.

Helping Infants Sleep

Because childhood sleep patterns vary, how you get your child to sleep depends in part on his age. The most dramatic changes in sleep occur during infancy. Whereas the typical newborn sleeps 80 percent of the time, by his first birthday he slumbers 55 percent of the time. For the first month the average infant briefly naps seven to eight times a day. By six weeks, however, he takes two to four slightly longer naps each day. At one year, babies usually indulge in two to three naps a day. Though all of these figures are mere averages they do reflect the enormous changes in the infant's sleep patterns.

As the child becomes acclimated to less sleep, he also discovers things about the world and about himself. During the first three months of life, the newborn is often startled by his own movements, which then keep him awake. Swaddling your child with a blanket—but not too tightly—will restrain these movements and enable him to doze off. Swaddling has the additional advantage of warming newborns. They can become extremely irritable and cold, and even turn blue, in an air-conditioned room or when lying next to a window on a chilly day.

Although their view has not been proven scientifically, many pediatricians believe that infants over three months of age are able to sleep better after an outdoor stroll. Whether this calms the child or whether it calms the parents, which in turn calms the child, remains unclear. Perhaps it's the fresh air.

If all else fails, taking your child for a brief drive usually does the trick. Maybe the regular motion of the car helps the infant snooze. Perhaps you're more relaxed, and therefore he's more relaxed. In any event, your mood and behavior do affect your child's sleep.

Ostensibly, parents raise children. But since children keep changing, parents are continually responding to their offspring's cues. By following these cues, mom and dad are being guided by their child on how to be a parent. The issue of who is raising whom during this first year contributes to a significant milestone—sleeping through the night, or *settling*.

By three months, about 70 percent of babies sleep continuously from midnight till dawn and an additional 13 percent do so by six months. Approximately 10 percent never sleep uninterruptedly during the first year. Physically traumatic births predispose infants to settling relatively late. On the other hand, sex, weight at birth, sleeping arrangements, and transient illnesses do not seem to affect the age at which a child settles. Half of already settled infants will subsequently wake up at night for several weeks.

Parents are often enraged at a child who, once settled, starts waking up again. What's more, mother and father may undeservedly blame themselves for being inadequate parents when this occurs. It's true that from the ages of three to twelve months, formerly settled infants who wake up again can be aggravated further by parental discord, anger, and anxiety. At other times, changes in sleeping arrangements, the arrival of a new sibling, a death in the family, and a marked alteration in mom's (and presumably dad's) emotional state can disrupt the infant's sleep. But in most cases, if the child's bodily needs are met, if he feels close to and secure with his parents, and if he's not overstimulated, his sleep problems will vanish quickly.

When your infant awakes screaming at night, rubbing his back, rocking him, or walking him about usually soothes him. Contrary to myth, carrying your child around in the middle of the night will not prolong his dependency on you.

Another myth is that pacifiers are harmful. Throughout their first year, infants derive gratification from sucking, even if they're wellfed. Pacifiers gratify infants, do not protract breast or bottle feeding, induce sleep, and are psychologically harmless.* They not only relax the child; they also give the mother and father some well-deserved time to themselves.

If you've tried all these measures and your baby still awakes hollering in the middle of the night, just let him *cry by himself.* Don't feel guilty about not rushing to his crib. After several nights of intermittent crying, he'll sleep through the night.

*Don't prop the bottle into the baby's mouth so that he'll suck himself to sleep. The relatively high carbohydrate concentration of most formulas will predispose teeth to cavities.

Helping Preschoolers Sleep

The child's next major sleep difficulty, which usually occurs during his second year, is a fear of going to sleep. Actually, it is less a fear of sleep and more a fear of losing his parents. This *separation anxiety* typically begins at eight to twelve months, peaks during the second and third years, and usually disappears by his fourth birthday. Occasionally, separation anxiety persists into the fourth year and beyond. It becomes painfully apparent when toddlers cry, fuss, or scream as soon as mom or dad leaves their sight. In their minds, if you're not visible, you don't exist; you've permanently abandoned them. In fact, discovering that things remain even though you can't see them, such as by playing peekaboo, is a major learning task for toddlers.

After you have tucked him into bed, his separation anxiety becomes obvious as he whines or screeches whenever you inch toward the door. At other times his fear will be less apparent: Perhaps he will look pathetic, saying, "my toes hurt" or "my legs don't work." Perhaps he will engage in diplomacy, by first negotiating to go to the bathroom, then demanding a glass of water, and then pleading for a story. All of these maneuvers are aimed at keeping you in his room. When you finally depart, and if he's able, he may follow you about like a stray puppy.

Initially, to quell his separation anxiety, you may have to indulge his requests for a trip to the potty or for a glass of water. You may wish to sit by him until he drifts off. All this requires patience. But as Ralph Waldo Emerson noted, "There never was a child so lovely but his mother was glad to get him to sleep." If while staying by his bed you convey that you're eager to leave, he may detect your discomfort, become increasingly anxious, and end up more alert than before.

When you decide that he should go to sleep without any shenanigans, try to hide whatever misgivings you might have. In a pleasant, matter-of-fact, but firm way, explain that he's already had his glass of water and trip to the john and that now it's time to sleep. Kiss him good night, and *without hesitation* leave the room. Of course he will cry; but at some point he will have to overcome separation anxiety. So will you. Don't drag out the process; get it over with. When your child's separation anxiety is mild, instead of slowly sneaking out of his room or repeatedly peeping inside it to check on him, once you've left for the night, don't return until morning. For both your and your child's sake, the short-term grief will be well worth the long-term gain.

Leaving your child with his favorite blanket or teddy bear can minimize his discomfort. They provide him with something familiar after you've departed and when he has to face the night alone. But don't force these objects onto your child; just make them available.

Following the *same* sleep-time routine, whether it's singing a lullaby, praying together, or reading a story, also provides the toddler with a feeling of security. When you take him on vacation, try to maintain this routine. Even though performing these rituals night after night may be a terrible bore to you, they leave your child better able to cope with separation anxiety and therefore with sleep.

You can also relieve separation anxiety by keeping his door open. The additional noise will not interfere with his sleep; it may, however, reduce his sense of isolation and confinement by allowing him to maintain contact with the "outside world."

During the latter half of his second year, your child's language skills accelerate. This development promotes sleep for two reasons. First, it enables the toddler to articulate and thereby to quell his anxiety. Babysitters often observe a kid initially scream when his parents go out for the evening, only to watch him later calm down after saying even something as rudimentary as "Mama, Dada, car." Second, if your child is bothered by something—a pain, a nightmare, or whatever—at least now he often can indicate the difficulty.

One of these problems is likely to be a fear of the dark. Although this common concern may arise during his second year, it is most profound during the third and fourth years. For some children, this fear may linger until their seventh or eighth birthday.

Going to bed alone in a dark room robs the child of the

familiar people and objects that afford him security. He can't see his crayon drawings, toy soldiers, nor even his chair. Instead, darkness enables frightening fantasies to replace reality. Ghosts and monsters, bears and gangsters fill the night void. Worse yet, he must confront these fantasies in what is essentially solitary confinement.

Although being able to have separate bedrooms for each child is a sign of affluence, bunking together reduces loneliness. With a favorite doll snuggled beneath his arm, and a brother or sister in the next bed, a child can face an eerie night with trusted companions. Having a radio on or sleeping with a toy also provides something familiar. Many youngsters want a night light; some feel secure only when all the bedroom lights are on. Though you may wonder how anybody can sleep with the lights on, it may be more pertinent to ask how children, with their fear of the dark, can sleep with the lights off.

Fear of death is also commonly associated with going to sleep. Four- to six-year-olds in particular are prone to confusing sleep and death. According to psychoanalysts, aggressive impulses often come to the fore during this period. Although disguised, thoughts of death and violence not uncommonly haunt their dreams and often lead to nightmares. For example, after her uncle died, five-year-old Lisa dreamed of flowers wilting in the family garden. On the same night, her six-year-old brother dreamed that a witch stole his dog, who was never seen again. After several nights and some parental reassurance, their sleep returned to normal.

Perhaps motivated by a fear of the dark, death, or separation from parents, some children try to sleep in the parental bed. They may also be curious to see what goes on there. Whatever the reason, the issue of allowing them to do so has been debated extensively, more often with theories than with facts. Psychiatrists regularly encounter patients who slept with one of their parents for fifteen or more years. (The record among my patients is held by a woman who slept with her father from the age of two until she ran away from home at the age of twenty-four.) Nevertheless, you should *not* conclude from such tales that a toddler should never be permitted to sleep alongside his parents. Psychiatrists see a select clientele; they do not treat the stable multitudes who as children occasionally climbed into their parents' bed. For centuries, out of necessity or design, children slept with their parents without suffering ill effects. Families that moved from one-room apartments into housing developments with private bedrooms were subsequently studied. After a period of sleeping apart, in which the children frequently awoke from nightmares, many families resumed sleeping together in a single room. Whether these children were responding adversely to sleeping alone or to changing homes remains unclear. Without adequate studies, we don't really know the consequences, favorable or unfavorable, of a youngster's sleeping beside his parents.

In the absence of proper research, it would seem reasonable to say that if a frightened child *occasionally* sleeps in your bed, it will not cause any harm. A child who knows that in an emergency his parents' bedroom is available for protection may feel sufficiently reassured to sleep by himself. Not everyone agrees with this position. Dr. Benjamin Spock, who is widely but mistakenly characterized as a proselytizer of permissiveness, states that children should *never* sleep in their parents' bed. He maintains that if your child crawls into your bed after a nightmare, you should "always bring him promptly and firmly back to his own bed." His chief concern is that once your child sleeps in your bed, you'll have a devil of a time getting him out of it. Although Dr. Spock's advice seems to be excessively rigid, his reservations deserve consideration. Wisely or not, our society encourages autonomy at an early age. Your child's sleeping *habitually* in your bed could interfere with his capacity to develop the independence that is so valued in our culture. It may also interfere with your own love life. After all, parents do have a right to privacy.

If your child is going to sleep in your bed, even if it's on a rare occasion, make sure that it is his rather than your needs that are being fulfilled. In many deteriorating marriages, a parent may sleep with his child to avoid sexual relations with his spouse. At other times parents who are afraid of being alone at night will encourage their child to sleep beside them. By projecting their feelings of loneliness or insecurity onto their child, these parents usually rationalize what they do by claiming their child "needs" them.

Even if they're in their own bed, children frequently do not fall asleep simply because they're not tired. Like adults, they should go to sleep when they're drowsy and not at some arbitrarily determined time. Very often, however, a child is too sleepy to be alert and too crabby to be asleep. When this happens, let him calm down during an open-ended quiet period, instead of coercing him to sleep. You can't *force* a child to sleep. All you can do, and that's quite a bit, is to create an atmosphere that facilitates sleep. Don't worry about his not getting sufficient rest. When his body needs sleep, he'll sleep.

Afternoon naps may postpone his nighttime sleepiness; if that happens, perhaps it's time to eliminate these naps. According to one study, the proportion of children who go without napping rises from 8 percent at age two to 12, 36, and 95 percent at ages three, four, and five, respectively. Granted, it's a relief to get Johnny "out of your hair" by sending him to bed at 2 P.M., but the same study demonstrates that many preschoolers get along fine without a nap.

Transient sleep problems are common among youngsters. They often occur after an overly stimulating day or in anticipation of some special event. When children, especially those aged two to four, go on vacation, are separated from a parent, or are admitted to the hospital, their sleep is likely to be disrupted. Don't worry about this temporary sleeplessness; it's all a normal part of growing up.

But as with children of all ages, if preschoolers suddenly display a decrease *or* increase of sleep that is marked and that continues for more than two weeks, the source of this change is worth investigating. If the problem is confined to sleep, then there's probably nothing to be concerned about. But if your child's persistent sleep difficulties coincide with the emergence of other symptoms, such as daytime fatigue, conflicts with playmates, phobias, despondency, or excessive misbehavior, he may be experiencing unusual psychological turmoil. If that's the case, consult your pediatrician or a child psychiatrist.

Helping School-age Children Sleep

Many school-age children, as well as preschoolers, need to calm down before going to sleep. It's ludicrous to expect a child to drop off immediately after roughhousing with dad. In order to "defuse" a youngster, some parents invoke a fifteen or twenty minute "quiet period" just before "lights out." During this time highly emotional and physical activities are forbidden, while reading, low-keyed games, and conversation are encouraged. The telling of an old-fashioned bedtime story can serve as a quiet period and affords a wonderful opportunity for togetherness and intimacy. There is also evidence that such story telling promotes language and reading skills.

Unfortunately, television watching is replacing story telling as a way to relax children at bedtime. Passively gazing at mesmerizing electronic visions may settle a child down, at least overtly. But many youngsters are unable to sleep after watching frightening TV programs, such as the recent spate of "disaster movies." After seeing *The Towering Inferno*, a seven-year-old repeatedly got out of bed and clung to her father's leg, fearing that their apartment would burst into flames. Research also indicates that some children who are calm while viewing television become agitated immediately afterwards, regardless of the program's content. Television is no substitute for the bedtime story. Reading him a story can soothe your child, forge bonds of closeness, and convey a sense of protection; television can do none of these things.

Just as television may be used as an electronic tranquilizer, a sleeping pill may inappropriately be used as a chemical tranquilizer. Some parents resort to hypnotic drugs even with their pediatrician's ill-advised consent. Although we don't know how frequently it occurs, this practice should be prohibited. Starting a child on these medications teaches poor sleep habits and invites future drug abuse. Most sleeping pills lose their effectiveness after several nights; using them can readily lead to psychological and often physical dependency (Chapter 9). Youngsters are especially apt to develop allergic side effects or to become agitated when given sleeping pills.

Children aged six to eight are frequently plagued by nightmares. But instead of tigers and sorcerers, teachers, parents, and friends inhabit their dreams. (Chapter 10 discusses how you can help your child with nightmares.) After the age of eight, however, nightmares appear much less often. By the age of eleven, they're quite unusual.

Some parents inadvertently contribute to their child's nightmares and difficulties in sleeping. Parents who dwell on their sleep tribulations or their horrendous nightmares unintentionally make their children feel obligated to solve these problems. Believing they are responsible, younger children may stay awake worrying about their distraught parent. They may also feel compelled to "protect" their parent by sleeping alongside him. Older children, in the process of identifying with their mother or father, may develop their parent's sleep-related symptoms. Saying she was a "chip off the old block," a patient confessed, "When I was seven, I so wanted to be like my father, I thought it was perfectly normal to stay awake half the night as he did." If your child is having difficulty sleeping, determine whether he's picking up some of your own concerns about sleep. Do his sleep problems resemble yours? Ask him how he feels about sleep; ask him what he thinks *you* feel about sleep. By discussing sleep, dreams, and nightmares with your child, you can clear up misconceptions and enable him to face the night without fear.

Helping Adolescents Sleep

According to psychoanalysts, adolescence is a period of intense psychological growth, change, and turmoil. After the onset of puberty, teenagers experience a reawakening of sexual impulses. They are likely to rebell against parental authority. Attempting to establish their own identities, they'll develop closer ties with friends, which some parents misinterpret as a lack of concern for them. The dreams of adolescents often reflect these psychological themes.

Their quest for independence may influence their sleep patterns. Wishing to do things *their* way, adolescents will go to bed when *they* want to and, on weekends, arise when *they* want to. Their sleep schedules are frequently erratic, especially when they're not attending school. They may sleep for three hours one night and twelve or more hours the next. All of this is normal adolescent behavior. As long as it doesn't interfere with their school, social, or work lives, it's best to leave well enough alone.

If it does interfere, it's time to have a serious but supportive chat with your son or daughter. Because of their desire to handle problems on their own, adolescents are often reluctant to admit to sleep problems. It may be up to you to initiate the conversation. Do so gently but firmly. Despite all his talk of independence, you're still his parent, and he still needs you. Don't abdicate your parental responsibilities under the guise of being a "modern" parent.

Most likely his sleep schedule has become derailed. When this happens, it's very difficult to get it back on the track. The suggestions advanced in Chapter 4, especially in the section entitled "Use Beds Only for Sleeping (Stimulus Control)" (pp. 77–80) are especially helpful for adolescents attempting to restore a normal sleep pattern.

It's common for them to have difficulties falling asleep. Their enthusiasm and energy for the following day's activities are likely to keep them up. As with adults, unless they're consistently fatigued during the day, don't worry about it (Chapter 3). Because teenagers rarely wake up in the middle of the night, we don't really know if this problem carries any special significance.

What is of concern is that a growing number of adolescents use drugs, especially alcohol, for "recreation" as well as for sleep. How to deal with this complex problem is beyond the scope of this book. But if drugs, whether legal or illegal, may be interfering with his or her sleep, you may wish to have your son or daughter read about them in Chapter 9.

If your teenager has been profoundly unhappy and has recently developed a distinctly altered sleep pattern, he might have a severe depression. Consistently disturbed sleep accompanied by extreme sadness or a pervasive lack of interest in life is among the first signs of a major depression. Because recent evidence shows a dramatic increase in adolescent suicide, depression among teenagers must be taken seriously. If a blood relative of yours has been depressed, you should be especially concerned, since depression runs in families.

But before you become too alarmed, remember that adolescents are frequently moody. If they don't make the football team, their lives are ruined. If so-and-so won't go out on a date with them, they'll threaten to become hermits. Normal adolescent moodiness must be distinguished from a major depression. Because depression has similar characteristics in both adults and teenagers, the sections on depression in Chapter 10 can help you decide whether your adolescent's unhappiness requires professional attention.

Preadolescent children can also suffer from depression. In addition, children of all ages can fall victim to a variety of other sleep disorders.

Childhood Sleep Disorders

A child's relatively immature psyche and soma render him highly susceptible to sleep disorders, especially to nightmares, night terrors, sleepwalking, sleep talking, head banging, and bed-wetting. These difficulties, and the painful memories of them, usually disappear with age. But at the time these symptoms are actually happening, the patience and imagination of the entire family are severely tested. Therefore, it's essential to know what to do about them.

Because adults suffer, albeit less frequently, from nightmares, night terrors, sleepwalking, and sleep talking, I've chosen to discuss these problems in Chapter 10. There I've also elaborated on narcolepsy, another sleep disorder, which often begins in adolescence and persists throughout life. Crib death, or the "sudden infant death syndrome," may sometimes be caused by sleep apnea, and is therefore reviewed in Chapter 10. Head banging and bed-wetting, however, occur almost exclusively during childhood.

The urge to bang a little sense into the head of a head banger is as universal as it is unnecessary. This weird behavior usually begins during the second half of a child's first year. As a prelude to sleep, he will rhythmically and often violently hit his head against a pillow or the crib. But despite the ferocity of head banging, the infant does not suffer any brain damage. At worst, he will bruise himself.

Why children bang their heads is largely a mystery. Among small children, head banging, by itself, is not caused by neurological disease, nor does it reflect an emotional disturbance. Instead, the rhythmic movements of the head banger, with their monotonous regularity, appear to be soothing to the baby. They also are a sign of the emerging musicality of the six-month-old—a valuable prerequisite for learning to speak and walk. Like thumb sucking, head banging seems to act as a comforter; both are benign habits that reduce tension, induce sleep, and go away naturally.

You should not restrain or scold the head banger. Just let him knock and rock about. To allay your own anxiety and to prevent a possible bruise, you may with so attach a canvas or prop a pillow against the crib's headboard. Otherwise, don't worry. If head banging persists beyond the age of one, however, consult a neurologist.

Bed-wetting (Enuresis)

Somewhere there is a former camp counselor I would like to thank. When I was eleven I eagerly departed for Camp Tanuga to spend my first summer away from home. After a week of playing baseball, hiking, and weaving ten dozen lanyard whistle chains, I was suddenly mortified. This counselor drew me aside and gently but directly told me that I had wet my bed for the past three nights. (I was so embarrassed, it never occurred to me why I had not discovered this for myself.) The counselor added that my bed-wetting would remain our secret and that many campers temporarily wet their beds. He also promised that before he went to sleep, he would awake me quietly and trot me off to the bathroom. He did so for several nights and my bed-wetting stopped. His simple yet sympathetic intervention spared me considerable shame and ridicule.

George Orwell was less fortunate. "I knew that bed-wetting was (a) wicked, and (b) outside my control. The second fact I was personally aware of, and the first I did not question. It was possible, therefore, to commit a sin without knowing you committed it, without wanting to commit it and without being able to avoid it."

To castigate a bed-wetting child is pointless and detrimental. Children do not wet their beds deliberately or out of sheer laziness. They no more wish to lie in urine-soaked sheets than you do. What's more, studies show that youngsters awakened after wetting their beds have no memory of being incontinent. Recent investigations have also disproven earlier psychoanalytic speculations that bed-wetting derives from unconscious hostility. In and of itself, bed-wetting is an innocuous and transient symptom. But the psychological scars induced by blaming or humiliating a child for bed-wetting are far more profound and enduring than the symptom itself. Most children outgrow bed-wetting, though it persists in 10 percent of seven-year-olds, 3 percent of twelve-year-olds, and 1 to 3 percent of seventeen- to twenty-eight-year-olds (army recruits).

There are two kinds of bed-wetting or enuresis (en-you-REE-sis). *Primary enuresis* is persistent bed-wetting past the ages of four or five, the time 85 to 90 percent of children have been toilet trained. Primary enuretics have never had a dry night's sleep. *Secondary enuresis* occurs in children who have already been trained and subsequently wet their beds.

Primary enuresis runs in families and has a genetic component. It may be caused by a delayed capacity to control the bladder or by a structural abnormality of the genito-urinary tract. Most often, however, expecting a child to be dry before he is neurologically able to be continent gives rise to needless concerns over bed-wetting.

Although secondary enuresis usually has psychological roots, it has been difficult to pinpoint what they are. Coercive toilet training has often been implicated, but never proven to cause bed-wetting. Contrary to psychiatric folklore, depression and anxiety have not been shown to produce enuresis; more likely, they are consequences of bed-wetting. Altering a child's environment—for example, by going on vacation or by starting school—triggers bed-wetting in some children but stops it in others. As a group, enuretics are more retiring, less confident, and more acquiescent than nonenuretics; with successful treatment, however, these traits reverse, suggesting they are results and not causes of bed-wetting. Children with major psychiatric disorders are more likely to be bed-wetters, but not vice versa. A study of 4,500 children showed that a youngster was apt to become enuretic later if between the ages of three and four, four or more of the following events occurred: (a) divorce or death in the family, (b) birth of a sibling, (c) moving, (d) hospitalization, (e) major accident, (f) surgery, or (g) separation of more than a month from the mother.* Whether these events directly caused subsequent bed-wetting or merely reflected general psychosocial distress leading to enuresis is unknown. It is clear, however, that children raised in poverty are more likely to become enuretic. It also remains a puzzle why boys, especially older ones, are more often enuretic than are girls. In sum, psychological factors play a major, though a still mysterious, role in enuresis.

Five percent of secondary enuretics have urinary-tract infections. The child may urinate more frequently, have a fever, or experience burning on urination; he may, however,

*Separation from the father does not seem to play a role in bed-wetting.

have none of these symptoms. On rare occasions diabetes causes enuresis.

Contrary to popular belief, dreams do not induce bed-wetting. It always occurs during NREM sleep, usually in the first third of the evening, and often *before* REM sleep ever begins. It starts in stage 4 and frequently continues when the child shifts into stages 2 or 1. If a child sleeps in a wet bed for several hours and is then awakened during a REM period, he may incorporate wetness into his dream. For example, an enuretic eight-year-old who wet his bed before having any REM sleep was later aroused from a dream in which friends threw him into a swimming pool.

If your child is enuretic, before you visit his pediatrician, try some simple but often effective measures:

• For three weeks reduce the amount of liquid he consumes after dinner. Stopping *all* fluids prior to bedtime may ensnare you in a power struggle with your child, who will then plead that he's "dying of thirst."

• Make sure that he goes to the bathroom immediately before going to sleep.

• Reward him by placing a star on a chart for every night he's dry. (This chart will also be a useful record for the pediatrician.) If your child gives you the go-ahead, show off his stars to the entire family.

• Without making a big to-do, congratulate him after every dry night. If he's dry for a week, you may wish to take him to the movies or perhaps buy him that special toy he's always wanted.

• A child who is old enough (about eight years or up), can set an alarm clock by himself that will go off before the time he usually wets. When it rings, he can go to the bathroom. In this way he can assume responsibility for and exert some control over his bed-wetting.

If these interventions don't work within three weeks, it's time to see the pediatrician.

Despite all the concerns over bed-wetting and the availability of effective remedies, relatively few parents actually seek medical help. Perhaps they're ashamed; perhaps they mistakenly believe that bed-wetting is a natural part of growing up; perhaps they're unaware that effective treatment exists. But whatever the reason, one study of eleven-year-old enuretics revealed that fewer than 30 percent were professionally evaluated or treated.

Many children cease wetting as soon as a doctor's appointment is made; others do so after they've visited the doctor but before treatment starts. When either of these occurs, some parents become angry at their child: "This only goes to show that if he really wanted to stop wetting, he could have." To these parents I can only respond, "So what? Maybe he just wanted to see if you were sufficiently concerned about him to make a doctor's appointment. Moreover, would you prefer that bed-wetting persist for months with treatment, or stop now without treatment?"

The pediatrician may recommend one of at least five approaches:

1. *Bell and Pad.* Sold by Sears, Roebuck and Company as the "wee alert," for thirty dollars, this device is safe and widely considered to be the best available treatment. Cure rates range from 60 to 100 percent. The bell and pad, also known as the "wee alarm," consists of a buzzer attached to a perforated metal or foil sheet on which the child sleeps. When he wets, the alarm goes off; through such conditioning, he eventually learns not to wet. Feeling that it embarrasses the child, some doctors object to this approach. I don't. If it's presented to the child in a favorable light, he will view it as an expression of parental concern. It certainly is less objectionable than bed-wetting. When this method does not work, it is usually because the gadget has not been installed properly or been used long enough. After the child has stopped wetting for two weeks, during which the child takes two pints of water nightly before retiring. By such "overlearning," the chance of relapse can be reduced threefold.

2. *Daytime training.* By rewarding a child for holding his urine for a progressively longer period each day, he is able to exert greater bladder control at night. After he feels the urge to void, he is to delay urinating in daily increments of

two to three minutes. Every time he succeeds, he receives a token *before* he goes to the bathroom. Later, after amassing enough tokens, he can exchange them for something he wants, like going to the circus. Daytime training is continued for twenty days or until he can delay urinating for forty-five minutes. Half the children who use this safe approach stop bed-wetting at night.

3. *Medications.* Small doses of Tofranil, an antidepressant drug (Chapter 9), will reduce the frequency of wetting in 85 percent and totally eliminate it in 30 percent of the cases. Despite its antidepressant activity, Tofranil alleviates enuresis not by altering the child's mood, but probably by affecting his bladder in ways that are currently not understood. Whereas the previously mentioned approaches take longer to work, Tofranil exerts its effect in a week. Once it is stopped, however, enuresis often re-emerges within three months. Antibiotics are prescribed when a urinary tract infection is causing the enuresis.

4. *Psychotherapy.* Psychotherapy is indicated only if the child has other emotional problems besides enuresis.

5. *Surgery.* Surgery may be helpful, but only in those unusual circumstances in which an abnormal bladder accounts for bed-wetting. If the doctor recommends an operation, before you proceed with it, make sure to obtain another opinion.

Childhood Insomnia

It's odd that children are plagued by almost every sleep problem except the one that is the greatest scourge of adults—insomnia. While still asleep, kids may stroll about the house, wet their beds, or awake with blood-curdling screams. But even with these difficulties, most children sleep sufficiently. Indeed, childhood insomnia is uncommon if you distinguish between the true child insomniac and the one who is merely recalcitrant at bedtime. Unlike the latter, the child insomniac is consistently tired during the day.

Except for the side effects of medication, developmental

or psychological problems usually account for childhood insomnia. For example, developmentally, toddlers normally pass through a stage of being obstinate; they may refuse to sleep, use the pot, eat, or walk. As a parent, you may take his stubbornness personally. Don't. Forcing him to sleep is useless and often provokes needless squabbles. Instead, just keep your cool; with time, he'll get over it. Psychologically, any major stressful event can precipitate insomnia—such as his starting school, getting a new sibling, or going on vacation. Being admitted to the hospital and experiencing family strife are other frequent causes of childhood sleeplessness.

Daytime overactivity can also lead to insomnia. Children with this difficulty usually fall into one of two extremes: they either rampage about because they have nothing to do or, being swamped with toys, they're unable to play constructively. But when a parent helps his child use his free time properly, normal sleep quickly returns.

Whatever the reason for your child's inability to sleep, if you're going to err, do so on the side of underplaying rather than overplaying the significance of his insomnia. Indeed, when he can't sleep, it's best to approach his problem with a sense of humor, but without being flip. Perhaps the end of the Lord Chancellor's song in Gilbert and Sullivan's *Iolanthe* ideally captures the proper spirit:

You're a regular wreck, with a crick in your neck, and no wonder you snore, for your head's on the floor, and you've needles and pins from your soles to your shins, and your flesh is a-creep, for your left leg's asleep, and you've cramp in your toes, and a fly on your nose, and some fluff in your lung, and a feverish tongue, and a thirst that's intense, and a general sense that you haven't been sleeping in clover;

But the darkness has passed, and it's daylight at last, and the night has been long—ditto ditto my song—and thank goodness they're both of them over!

APPENDICES

APPENDIX A

Sleep Disorders Centers

In recent years the number of sleep disorders centers has increased dramatically. So although I've tried to make this list of sleep clinics as comprehensive as possible, any such roster will inevitably be somewhat out of date. If this list does not mention a clinical sleep disorders center in your area, I'd suggest calling the department of psychiatry at the closest medical school or hospital for the name of the nearest sleep laboratory. An alternative way to obtain the name of the closest sleep clinic is to contact the Association of Sleep Disorders Centers, c/o Dr. Merrill M. Mitler, Sleep Disorders Center, Department of Psychiatry, SUNY at Stony Brook, Stony Brook, N.Y., 11794 (516) 246-2561.

Whereas some sleep disorders centers exclusively conduct research, others perform research *and* provide diagnostic and treatment services. This roster of sleep laboratories in the United States and Canada includes only those that offer evaluation and treatment.

You should check whether the cost of an assessment in a sleep clinic is covered by your health-insurance policy. If your sleep problems are not resolved by the program outlined in this book, however, an evaluation by the staff of a sleep disorders center is certainly well worth the money.

Although some sleep laboratories will see self-referred patients, others require an initial referral from your physician. Those clinics wishing a doctor's referral are indicated by an asterisk (*).

ALABAMA

University of Alabama Sleep
  Laboratory
University Station, University
  of Alabama
Birmingham, Alabama 35294
205–934–3636
Vernon Pegram, Ph.D.

ARKANSAS

Sleep Disorders Clinic*
University of Arkansas for
  Medical Sciences
4301 West Markham
Little Rock, Arkansas 72205
501–661–5166
Edgar Lucas, Ph.D.

CALIFORNIA

Sleep Disorders Center*
Holy Cross Hospital
15031 Rinaldi Street
Mission Hills, California,
  91345
213–365–8051 Ext. 1497
Elliott R. Phillips, M.D.

Sleep Disorders Center
University of California Irvine
  Medical Center
101 City Drive South
Orange, California, 92668
714–634–5777
Jon Sassin, M.D.
NOTE: Doctor's referral
  preferred

Sleep Disorders Clinic*
Department of Psychiatry,
  V.A. Hospital
3350 La Jolla Village Drive
San Diego, California, 92161
714–453–3436
Daniel Kripke, M.D.
NOTE: Only for veterans from
  the San Diego area

Sleep Disorders Center
Suite 1402
1260 15th Street
Santa Monica, California, 90404
213–451–3270
John Beck, M.D.

Sleep Disorders Center*
Stanford University Medical
  Center
Stanford, California, 94305
415–497–6601
*William C. Dement, M.D.,
  Ph.D.*

Stanford Sleep Disorders
  Clinics*
Stanford University Medical
  Center
Stanford, California, 94305
415–497–7548
Laughton Miles, M.D., Ph.D.

COLORADO

Sleep Laboratory*
National Jewish Hospital and
  Research Center/National
  Asthma Center
3800 East Colfax Avenue
Denver, Colorado, 80206
303–388–4461 Ext. 332
David W. Shucard, Ph.D.
David W. Hudgel, M.D.

FLORIDA

Sleep Disorders Center
Mount Sinai Hospital
4300 Alton Road
Miami Beach, Florida, 33140
305–674–2613
Lawrence Scrima, Ph.D.

ILLINOIS

Sleep Disorders Center*
Suite 214, Wesley Pavilion
Northwestern Memorial
  Hospital
Northwestern University
  Medical Center
250 East Superior Street
Chicago, Illinois, 60611
312–649–2650
Juan J. Cayaffa, M.D.

Sleep Disorders Service and
  Research Center
Rush-Presbyterian-St. Luke's
  Hospital
1753 West Congress Parkway
chicago, Illinois, 60612
312–942–5440
Rosalind Cartwright, Ph.D.

Clinical Neurophysiology
  Unit*
University of Chicago School
  of Medicine
950 East 59th Street
Chicago, Illinois, 60637
312–947–6093
J. P. Spire, M.D.

LOUISIANA

Sleep Disorders Center
Department of Psychiatry and
  Neurology
Tulane Medical School
New Orleans, Louisiana, 70112
504–588–5236
John Goethe, M.D.

MARYLAND

Sleep Disorders Center of The
  Johns Hopkins University
Baltimore City Hospital
Baltimore, Maryland, 21224
301–396–8603
Richard Allen, M.D., Ph.D.

MASSACHUSETTS

Sleep Laboratory and Sleep
  Center
Boston State Hospital
591 Morton Street
Boston, Massachusetts, 02124
617–734–1300 Ext. 208
Ernest Hartmann, M.D.

Laboratory of Neurophysiology
Massachusetts Mental Health
  Center
25 Shattuck Street
Boston, Massachusetts, 02115
617–734–1300 Ext. 208
Allan Hobson, M.D.

Sleep Clinic
Peter Bent Brigham Hospital
721 Huntington Avenue
Boston, Massachusetts, 02115
617–732–6750
Quentin Regestein, M.D.

Sleep Disorders Program
The Children's Hospital
  Medical Center
300 Longwood Avenue
Boston, Massachusetts, 02115
617–734–6000 /Ext. 3988 or
  2071
Myron Belfer, M.D.
NOTE: Only for those under the
  age of twenty–one

Sleep and Wake Disorder Unit
Department of Neurology
University of Massachusetts
  Medical Center
Worcester, Massachusetts,
  01605
617–856–2661
Sheldon Kapen, M.D.

MICHIGAN

Sleep Disorders Center
Henry Ford Hospital
2799 West Grand Boulevard
Detroit, Michigan, 48202
313–876–2233
Thomas Roth, Ph.D.

MINNESOTA

Minnesota Regional Sleep
  Disorders Center
Hennepin County Medical
  Center
701 Park Avenue South
Minneapolis, Minnesota, 55415
612–347–6288
Milton Ettinger, M.D.

NEW HAMPSHIRE

Sleep Disorders Center*
Department of Psychiatry,
  Dartsmouth Medical School
Hanover, New Hampshire,
  03755
603–646–2043
Michael Sateia, M.D.
NOTE: Diagnostic services only

NEW JERSEY

Sleep/Wake Studies
College of Medicine and
    Dentistry of New Jersey–New
    Jersey Medical School
100 Bergen Street
Newark, New Jersey, 07103
James Minard, Ph.D.
NOTE: Patients are requested to
    write for appointments.

NEW YORK

Sleep Disorders Center
Department of Psychiatry,
    Albany Medical College
75 New Scotland Avenue
Albany, New York, 12208
518–445–6851
Vincenzo Castaldo, M.D.

Sleep-Wake Disorders Center
Montefiore Hospital
111 East 210th Street
Bronx, New York, 10467
212–920–4841
Elliot D. Weitzman, M.D.

Sleep Laboratory*
Columbia-Presbyterian
    Medical Center
630 West 168th Street
New York, New York, 10032
212–694–5341
New Kavey, M.D.

Sleep Disorders Center*
Department of Psychiatry,
    SUNY at Stony Brook
Stony Brook, New York, 11794
516–246–2561
Merrill M. Mitler, Ph.D.

OHIO

Sleep Disorders Center
26900 Cedar Road
Beachwood, Ohio, 44122
216–464–5330
Herbert Weiss, M.D.

Sleep Disorders Center
University of Cincinnati
    Hospital
Cincinnati General Division
Mont Reid Pavilion, Room 23
234 Goodman Avenue
Cincinnati, Ohio, 45267
513–872–5087
Milton Kramer, M.D.

Sleep Disorders Center
Mount Sinai Hospital
University Circle
Cleveland, Ohio, 44106
216–421–3732
Herbert Weiss, M.D.

Sleep Disorders Center
St. Lukes Hospital
11311 Shaker Boulevard
Cleveland, Ohio, 44104
216–368–7000
Joel Steinberg, M.D.

Sleep Disorders Evaluation
  Center
Ohio State University Hospitals
410 West 10th Avenue
Columbus, Ohio, 43210
614–421–8260
Helmut S. Schmidt, M.D.

OKLAHOMA

Sleep Disorders Center*
Presbyterian Hospital
13th and Lincoln Boulevards
Oklahoma City, Oklahoma,
  73104
405–271–6312
William Orr, Ph.D.

PENNSYLVANIA

Sleep Disorders Center
Western Psychiatric Institute
  and Clinic
3811 O'Hara Street
Pittsburgh, Pennsylvania,
  15261
412–624–2246
David Kupfer, M.D.
NOTE: Doctor's referral
  preferred

Sleep Disorders Center
Crozer-Chester Medical Center
15th Street and Upland Avenue
Upland-Chester, Pennsylvania,
  19013
215–874–1233
Calvin R. Stafford, M.D.

TENNESSEE

Baptist Memorial Hospital
  Sleep Disorders Center*
899 Madison Avenue
Memphis, Tennessee, 38146
901–522–5651
Helio Lemmi, M.D.

TEXAS

Sleep Disorders Center
Metropolitan Professional
  Building
1303 McCullough
San Antonio, Texas, 78212
512–223–4026
J. Catesby Ware, Ph.D.
Philip J. Moorad, M.D.

Sleep Facility*
Clinical Psychophysiology
  Laboratory
Audie Murphy Memorial V.A.
  Hospital
7400 Merton Minter Boulevard
San Antonio, Texas, 78284
512–696–9660 Ext. 6525
Augustin de la Peña, Ph.D.

Sleep Facility
Behavioral Medicine
  Laboratory
Department of Psychiatry,
  UTHSCSA
7703 Floyd Curl Drive
San Antonio, Texas, 78284
512–691–7315
Johnnie G. Fisher, M.D.

Sleep Disorders Center*
Baylor College of Medicine
Houston, Texas, 77030
713–790–4886
Ismet Karacan, M.D.

CANADA

Sleep Disorders Investigation
    and Research Unit*
Ottawa General Hospital
43 Bruyère Street
Ottawa, Ontario, K1N 5C8
613–231–4738
Robert Broughton, M.D.
NOTE: Evaluation only

Sleep Disorders Clinic*
Toronto Western Hospital
399 Bathurst Street
Toronto, Ontario, M5T 2S8
416–369–5109
Harvey Moldofsky, M.D.

Center of Studies on
    Sleep Polysomnography
    Laboratory*
Hôpital du Sacre-Coeur
5400 ouest, Boulevard Gouin
Montreal, Quebec, H4J 1C5
514–333–2692
Jacques Montplaisir, M.D.
John Walsh, Ph.D.

APPENDIX B

Progressive Relaxation Instructions

While conducting progressive relaxation, you may prefer listening to tape-recorded instructions instead of recalling the directions by yourself. Using a tape recording may enable you to concentrate fully on relaxation without being distracted by having to remember the instructions.

The person you choose to tape record these instructions should be somebody you trust and whose voice will calm you. This person could be your spouse, a relative, a friend, or even yourself. Whoever it is should practice reading this transcript before making a recording. During these rehearsals you or the reader might wish to add or delete phrases or to alter the speed and intonations of the recitation. The pauses in the transcript serve merely as guidelines for the reader. Make a recording that best suits your particular needs. Since your goal for learning progressive relaxation is to facilitate sleep, the relaxation portions of these directions should be recited soothingly.

To create an optimal final recording I'd recommend initially recording a practice recitation. Because "live" voices sound different from taped ones, you should first hear how the recitation sounds on tape. If after you make a "final" taped version, you're dissatisfied with it, record another one. Settle only for a tape that is suitably soporific.

Chapter 5 indicates that there are numerous ways to perform progressive relaxation. The following transcript is one approach; it starts with a total-body muscular contraction and ends with total-body relaxation. You might wish to record another set of instructions based on your current needs and preferences.

Transcript of Instructions

"Begin by getting as comfortable as you can. Unloosen any tight-fitting clothes (five-second pause). Position yourself comfortably with your limbs uncrossed (ten-second pause).

"Note the tension in your body (five-second pause). Now, gently close your eyes (three-second pause). Observe that this tension decreases slightly when your eyes are closed (five-second pause).

"Now, take in a deep breath and hold it (five-second pause), and then calmly breathe out. Just let the air out quite automatically. Enjoy the wave of relaxation that flows throughout your body (ten-second pause).

"Now, (read with emphasis) contract *all* the muscles in your body. Squeeze them as tightly as you possibly can...and then make them even tighter. Your *entire* body, from your head to your toes, should feel like a steel rod (three-second pause).

"Now, *suddenly* release all your muscles; (with a quieter and calmer voice) let them relax fully and totally. Contrast your former tenseness with the pleasant and growing experience of relaxation (five-second pause). Simply concentrate on relaxation. Feel the tension spreading from the top of your head straight through the tips of your toes (five-second pause).

"Let your right arm relax completely. If you wish to shake it a bit to relax further, go right ahead. Just let your right forearm, arm, hand, and fingers lose all of their tension (three-second pause). Similarly, make sure your entire left arm is fully relaxed. Allow all of the tension to drain out of it. Shake it about to release any residual tension. Enjoy the feeling of becoming increasingly relaxed (five-second pause).

"As your entire body relaxes, let all your face muscles relax. Your forehead muscles are relaxing and the muscles around your nose are relaxing. The loss of tension is spreading throughout your face. As you breathe, you can feel the air gently streaming in and then out of your nostrils. Relax the muscles around your mouth; as you do so, your mouth may open slightly. Relax your tongue so that it gently rests on the bottom of your mouth. Release all the tension from your cheeks . . . and then from your lips . . . and then from your jaw and chin muscles. Just relax (five-second pause).

"As you relax, breathe comfortably; you will begin to feel increasingly and totally relaxed, tranquil, and serene. If your mind starts to wander, that's okay, Just refocus on relaxation.

"Your neck and throat muscles are now relaxing more than before. Eliminate any kinks in your neck. If you wish to swallow at any time, go ahead (five-second pause). Just relax the muscles on the sides and the back of your neck as fully as possible (five-second pause).

"Let the tension in your chest dissipate totally (five-second pause). Continue to breathe naturally and pleasantly. When you breathe out, relax your stomach so that your belly feels soft like jelly. Continue to breathe comfortably (three-second pause), and with each breath feel yourself sinking into a deeper and deeper state of relaxation (ten-second pause).

"Relax your buttocks and hips (five-second pause). Feel the relaxation spread to your legs. Wiggle your toes to relax them further. Let all the tension in your right leg flow out of your right thigh . . . calf . . . foot . . . and toes. Relax your entire right leg (five-second pause). Now, let your entire left leg become completely and totally relaxed. Check to see that all the lingering tension in your left thigh . . . calf . . . foot . . . and toes disappears (five-second pause).

"Review every muscle group to rid them of any remaining tension. Your arms . . . face . . . neck . . . throat . . . chest . . . stomach . . . buttocks . . . hips . . . and leg muscles. Enjoy the calm and serenity of relaxation (ten-second pause).

"To further deepen your relaxation, every time you breathe out, you'll notice all of your muscles becoming heavier. Each one is feeling heavier and heavier every time you exhale (five-second pause). Inhale (five-second pause), and then, as you exhale, feel your muscles becoming heavier and more relaxed (five-second pause). Enjoy this wonderful experience of complete relaxation (ten-second pause).

"Every time you exhale you'll notice your muscles becoming even heavier as a sense of blissful tranquility prevails (five-second pause). Check to see if any tension still resides anyplace in your body (five-second pause). If so, let it gently slip away (five-second pause). Your muscles are now relaxed and heavy (five-second pause).

"Continue to breathe naturally. But now when you exhale, you'll also feel yourself descending into a deeper state of restfulness. Imagine yourself on a cloud, gently floating downwards from the sky; the farther down you go, the sleepier you become (ten-second pause). Don't force sleepiness; let your body do it for you. Your heavy muscles are slowly pulling the cloud down and down and down, as you feel sleepier, and sleepier, and sleepier. Don't force yourself to be sleepy. Just let it happen. With every breath you will naturally become tired. Feel your mind and body slowing down (ten-second pause). Every time you breathe out you'll become sleepier and sleepier (ten-second pause).

"And sleepier (ten-second pause).

"And sleepier (ten-second pause).

"With each breath you'll continue to drift deeper . . . and deeper . . . and deeper . . . to sleep."

APPENDIX C

Additional Readings

There are many scientifically accurate and at the same time highly readable books that convey to a general audience the richness of and fascination with sleep, its disorders, and treatment. I particularly recommend the following:

Dement, William C. *Some Must Watch While Some Must Sleep*. San Francisco: W. H. Freeman, 1974.

Diamond, Edwin. *The Science of Dreams*. Garden City, N.Y.: Doubleday, 1962.

Foulkes, David. *The Psychology of Sleep*. New York: Charles Scribner's Sons, 1966.

Hartmann, Ernest L. *The Functions of Sleep*. New Haven: Yale University Press, 1973.

Hartmann, Ernest L. *The Sleeping Pill*. New Haven: Yale University Press, 1978.

Hauri, Peter. *The Sleep Disorders*. Kalamazoo, Mich.: Upjohn, 1977.

Kleitman, Nathaniel. *Sleep and Wakefulness*. Rev. ed.; Chicago: University of Chicago Press, 1963.

Luce, Gay Gaer, and Segal, Julius, *Insomnia: The Guide for Troubled Sleepers*. Garden City, N.Y.: Doubleday, 1968.

Luce, Gay Gaer, and Segal, Julius. *Sleep: The Third World of the Mind!* New York: Arena, 1975.

Oswald, Ian. *Sleep*. Middlesex, England: Penguin, 1966.

Webb, Wilse B. *Sleep: The Gentle Tyrant*. Englewood Cliffs, N.J.: Prentice-Hall, 1975.

Index